PRACTICAL
MEDITATION

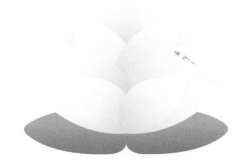

PRACTICAL
MEDITATION

GIOVANNI DIENSTMANN

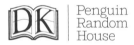
Penguin
Random
House

Editor Alice Horne
Senior Art Editor Karen Constanti
Designer Emma Forge
Senior Jacket Creative Nicola Powling
Jackets Coordinator Lucy Philpott
Producer (Pre-Production) Rebecca Fallowfield,
Luca Frassinetti
Senior Producer Ché Creasey
Creative Technical Support Sonia Charbonnier
Managing Editor Dawn Henderson
Managing Art Editor Marianne Markham
Art Director Maxine Pedliham
Publishing Director Mary-Clare Jerram

Illustrations Keith Hagan

First published in Great Britain in 2018
by Dorling Kindersley Limited
80 Strand, London, WC2R 0RL

A CIP catalogue record for this book
is available from the British Library.
ISBN: 978-0-2413-3167-5

CONTENTS

THE MANY TYPES OF MEDITATION

INTEGRATING AND DEEPENING

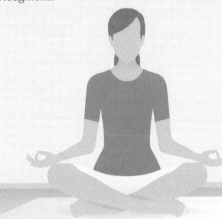

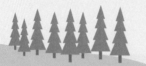

FOREWORD

In an age when we're always "switched on", it can be especially difficult to shake off stress and negative emotions, stick to our goals, or really focus on what is happening in the present moment. It can seem as though life is passing by without us noticing, and we may even find ourselves feeling far away from the person we want to be. If that sounds familiar, you've come to the right place: meditation can help you address all these concerns, and many more. By picking up this book, you have already taken an important step towards a calmer, more contented life.

Meditation has been an essential part of my life since I was 14 years old. I was a very restless, anxious, and angry person, really in need of meditation, but that is not why I started meditating. I started meditating in search of a deeper meaning in life, self-mastery, and the actualization of the human potential. I was deeply fascinated with the mystical and the spiritual, so I read everything I could get my hands on and visited every teacher I could. These foundational years of learning are distilled into **chapter 1** of this book, where you'll begin your journey by discovering what meditation is, its proven benefits, and what it can do for your life.

In **chapter 2**, you'll bring some immediate calm to your life with a first taste of meditation and five "mini-meditations" which will help you to identify which techniques could work for you. You'll also gain clarity about what to expect from your practice and how to avoid common pitfalls on the way.

I've now meditated every day for over 18 years. This has radically transformed my mind and experience of the world, especially as a result of some key awakenings in my journey. With these "points of no return", I found that many negative thought- and emotional patterns disappeared almost entirely, and any sizeable psychological suffering no longer lasts more than 5 minutes. None of this could have happened without a well-established daily meditation practice. A daily commitment doesn't need to be daunting: in **chapter 3** you'll find out how to start your practice in a way that is sustainable and rewarding. You'll learn how to build meditation as a habit and how to overcome some common obstacles you might face as a beginner meditator.

In my intense search of personal growth and enlightenment, I have experimented with over 80 styles of meditation. From these, I have selected 39 of the most popular and accessible techniques from the main traditions to feature in **chapter 4**, all of which you can practise at home in simple steps.

It took me many years, hundreds of books, hours of reflection, and countless practice sessions to finally connect all the pieces of the meditation puzzle. **Chapter 5** is where all of this pays off: here, you'll discover how to integrate meditation into your life and how to use it to deal with day-to-day challenges, such as negative emotions, problem solving, and how to improve performance in areas from your career to sport. You'll also learn how to take your practice to the next level.

This is the book I wish existed when I started my journey, as it would have saved me so much time and energy. You can open it at any page and be sure that you will learn something useful and practical. Or, you can gain a broad understanding of everything you need to know by reading it from cover to cover.

It's now time to pause for a second. Feel into your body. Take a deep breath. And turn the page. May your journey into meditation be transformative!

Giovanni Dienstmann
Meditation teacher, author, and coach

UNDERSTANDING
MEDITATION

WHAT IS MEDITATION?

Starting from the ground up

Meditation was originally created to overcome suffering, find a deeper meaning in life, and connect to a higher reality. Today, it is also used to find personal growth, improve performance, and achieve optimal health and wellbeing.

Meditation is an exercise for your mind – a type of contemplative practice. This exercise takes different shapes depending on the style of meditation that you are practising but, in general, it involves:

● **Relaxation.** Relaxing your body, slowing your breath, and calming your mind.

● **Stillness.** Traditionally, meditation involves stilling the body, either in a seated or lying-down position. However, some techniques are more dynamic, such as Kinhin (walking meditation).

● **Looking inside.** Whether you keep your eyes open or closed, meditation turns your attention inwards, towards yourself, rather than towards the external world.

● **Awareness.** In meditation, you become a witness to your mental and emotional states, and let go of thoughts, feelings, and distractions.

● **Focus.** Most practices involve focusing the attention on a single object, such as a candle flame or your breath (concentration), while others focus the attention on noticing whatever shows up in your consciousness in the present moment (observation).

By nature, certain techniques incorporate a spiritual element – their goal is to help the practitioner to experience altered states of consciousness and realities beyond the material world. However, most meditations can be practised in a secular way, so you don't need to believe or follow any particular religion or philosophy. This secular approach is the one followed in this book.

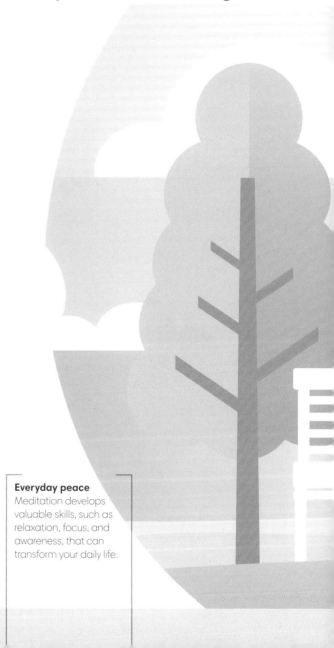

Everyday peace
Meditation develops valuable skills, such as relaxation, focus, and awareness, that can transform your daily life.

10

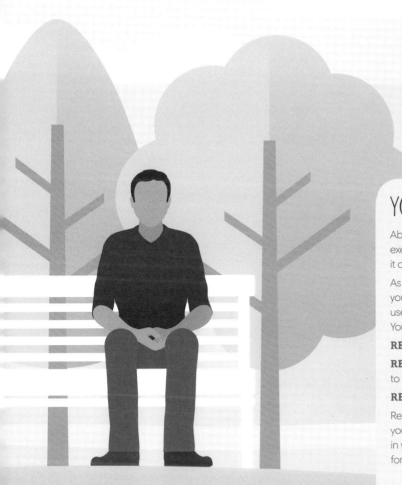

"Meditation expands your horizons in life, showing you options you didn't even know existed."

YOUR JOURNEY

Above all, meditation is a way to understand, exercise, and explore your mind. This makes it a deeply personal experience.

As each chapter in this book guides you on your journey of self-exploration, you may find it useful to keep a journal about your experiences. You can use it as a space to:

REFLECT on your experiences and feelings.

REINVIGORATE your practice by referring to your aims when you lack motivation.

REMIND yourself how far you have come.

Remember that there is no final destination in your journey: as you learn more and advance in your practice, you will find more opportunities for personal growth and development.

MEDITATION MYTH BUSTING

Common questions and misconceptions

As you start your meditation journey, it's normal to have lots of questions about the practice, or even about what exactly meditation is. Getting to know a bit more about it and dispelling some widespread myths will open up your path of discovery.

Q DOES MEDITATION REALLY WORK?
Meditation is an ancient practice that has been helping people to be happier, more peaceful, and to live better lives for millennia (see pp.16–19). Its many benefits to your mind and body have now been proven by science (see pp.22–27).

Q IS MEDITATION RELIGIOUS?
Though some techniques are religious by nature, meditation itself is an exercise for your mind. As long as you follow secular techniques, you don't need to hold any particular beliefs, so it does not conflict with any religion, nor does it conflict with atheism.

Q IS MEDITATION THE SAME AS MINDFULNESS?
No – mindfulness can be taken to mean a number of different things. For example, mindfulness can be a practice of following the breath, or of observing whatever is arising in your present moment experience. Taken in this way, mindfulness is one of many types of meditation (see pp.82–83). On the other hand, mindfulness can also refer to the qualities of awareness, remembrance, and watchfulness. In this sense, mindfulness is a skill involved in all types of meditation and which can be practised in many daily life activities (see pp.140–141).

Q ARE TAI CHI AND YOGA FORMS OF MEDITATION?
Tai Chi and Yoga are forms of body-mind exercises that have a contemplative component to them. While they are not exactly forms of meditation on their own, they can enhance your practice and can be performed with a meditative spirit (see pp.96–97 and pp.94–95). They also share some benefits with meditation as they are slow and mindful by nature.

Q DO I NEED A CALM MIND IN ORDER TO MEDITATE?
No. Just as you don't need to be strong to go to the gym, you don't need a certain state of mind to be able to meditate. Meditation helps you achieve calmness of mind.

"Having an open and curious mind helps you get the most out of your meditation practice."

Q IS MEDITATION DIFFICULT?

As a process, meditation is simple and anyone can practise it. The state of meditation, as it is traditionally defined, is more difficult to achieve and happens only when the mind is perfectly focused on a single object. However, very few people achieve this consistently, and you can still access the many benefits of meditation without it.

Q DO I NEED TO STOP OR EMPTY MY MIND IN MEDITATION?

You cannot stop your mind as an act of will. Instead, in meditation you intently focus your mind on one thing to the exclusion of all others (see pp.74–75). As your mind becomes fully engaged in one thing,

your thinking is redirected and your mind becomes quiet and still. However, it can take years of practice to achieve this state, so it is not something that you need to consider in the beginning.

Q IS MEDITATION ALL ABOUT RELAXATION AND LIVING IN THE MOMENT?

Relaxation and present moment awareness are crucial to meditation – without them you cannot truly meditate – but these are just the first steps. Depending on which technique you follow, meditation also applies your mind in different ways to develop awareness, focus, introspection, and insight. Meditation starts with relaxation, but is ultimately an exercise to help you better understand, control, and expand your mind.

Q IS THERE A RIGHT OR WRONG WAY TO MEDITATE?

Just as there are right and wrong ways to exercise or eat well, there are specific techniques that need to be followed in meditation, which unfold into particular experiences and stages of practice. Without proper guidance, you may experience some relaxation through meditation, but you will make no progress beyond that point.

13

MEDITATION MYTH BUSTING

CONTINUED ▶

UNDERSTANDING MEDITATION

14

Q IS DEEP RELAXATION IN MEDITATION LIKE SLEEP?

In deep sleep there is total unawareness, whereas meditation is a state of heightened awareness. Meditation also helps you to relax consciously and develop your focus, while sleep simply gives you rest and restoration.

Q IS IT SELF-INDULGENT TO SPEND TIME MEDITATING?

No. Like sleeping and eating, meditating is essential to staying healthy, balanced, and well. Only when you are in your best state can you truly serve others and engage in unselfish activities effectively, without burning out. The positive state of mind you achieve from meditation will be greatly beneficial to those around you.

Q IS MEDITATION A WAY TO RUN AWAY FROM LIFE?

Quite the opposite: distraction is a way of running away from life. Meditation cuts away all distraction and places you in front of yourself. Meditation also teaches you to arrive at a state that is deeper than all your problems. While some people may want to use this as an escape strategy, that is not what meditation itself teaches.

Q WILL MEDITATION MAKE ME SLOW, APATHETIC, AND PASSIVE?

No, but your attitude towards the practice and the philosophies around it might have this effect on you. Meditation gives you tranquillity and creates more pause and clarity in your life. You will become less restless and less dominated by your emotions. This may make you appear different in the eyes of others, but in reality, the skills developed through meditation enhance your ability to act wisely and effectively in life.

Q DO I NEED TO BURN INCENSE, CHANT "OM", AND WEAR SPECIAL CLOTHES?

No. Some people do find it useful to establish some form of ritual around their practice as this can help to ground and focus the mind (see pp.164–165), but this is not essential to the process of meditation itself.

Q DO I NEED TO SIT IN A SPECIAL POSTURE IN ORDER TO MEDITATE?

Specific seated postures are recommended for most meditation techniques, as they can have a powerful effect on your state of mind. You can choose from several variations to suit your needs (see pp.66–69).

Q DO I NEED TO CLOSE MY EYES TO MEDITATE?

Not always. Closing your eyes helps you to focus your attention inwards, but some meditation techniques, such as Zazen (see pp.84–85) and Trataka (see pp.102–103), are done with your eyes open, which has the advantage of helping you to be more present and alert.

Q HOW SHOULD I CHOOSE A MEDITATION TECHNIQUE?

There is no single style of meditation that is superior to all others. Different approaches work for different people – it is simply a matter of experimenting with different techniques and seeing which work best for you. This will also depend on your goals for the practice (see pp.80–81), so it helps to gain clarity around what you seek from meditation first. Bear in mind that as your needs and goals change in life, you may find that you will benefit from different techniques at different times.

Q HOW LONG SHOULD I MEDITATE FOR?

It depends on the benefits you seek and how interested you are in the practice, but it is generally best to start small. Don't overstretch your motivation to practise; instead increase the length of your session as you feel the need (see pp.58–61).

Q HOW OFTEN SHOULD I MEDITATE?

To get the most out of meditation, you need to meditate every day, ideally at the same time and in the same place (see pp.58–61). You can also introduce meditation and meditative activites into your daily life (see pp.140–141).

Q DO I NEED A MEDITATION TEACHER?

You don't need a teacher to get started with meditation, especially if you primarily seek its health and wellbeing benefits. But as your practice deepens, you may feel you need more guidance. A teacher can help improve your technique, tackle obstacles (see pp.166–167), and build meditation more fully into your life (see pp.140–141).

"The best mindset for meditation is one of non-judgment, curiosity, patience, and perseverance."

A QUESTIONING MINDSET

Having an open and questioning mind is an important part of meditation. For example:

AWARENESS. Meditation invites you to ask yourself how your body is feeling, what state your mind is in, and to question thoughts and actions that are usually automatic. This develops greater awareness, a crucial skill in meditation.

THE BIGGER QUESTIONS. Meditation encourages us to ask difficult questions, such as "Who am I?" and "What is the meaning of life?"

GOING DEEPER. By fostering curiosity around your practice – researching more about it, or asking a meditation teacher questions – you will connect more deeply with meditation.

MEDITATION TRADITIONS

A global timeline

Meditation developed over many centuries in several philosophical traditions, adapting for the different and changing needs of its practitioners. This timeline shows the key dates in its development according to the main traditions.

 YOGA
C.1,500 BCE

The oldest written evidence of meditation appears in ancient Hindu scripture, known as the Vedas, which is also linked to the Yogic tradition. The Yogic tradition is still alive and thriving, with hundreds of lineages or schools including the modern Yoga movement (Hatha Yoga), which emphasizes postures (asanas) and breathing exercises.

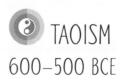 TAOISM
600–500 BCE

The Chinese sage Laozi establishes Taoism in China. Taoism seeks to get rid of artificialities, find harmony with nature (*Tao*), cultivate energy (*qi*), balance yin and yang, and achieve immortality. Taoists develop many meditation practices over the centuries, including Tai Chi, simplified forms of which are popular today. However, more esoteric techniques remain unknown outside Taoist circles.

5,000 BCE	3,000 BCE	1,500 BCE	600 BCE

 YOGA
C.5,000–3,500 BCE

Wall art depicting people seated in meditative postures with half-closed eyes appears in the Indus Valley, South Asia. This is one of the earliest pieces of evidence of meditation and has been linked to the Hindu tradition, which includes both the Yogis, who meditated in caves, and the sages of the Vedic culture.

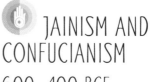 JAINISM AND CONFUCIANISM
600–400 BCE

Jainism, which focuses on non-violence and self-denial, is founded in India by Mahavira; and Confucianism, a society-centred philosophy, in China by Confucius. Both develop approaches to meditation, such as Preksha Dhyana (Soul Insight) and Quiet Sitting (*Jingzuo*). Though they still exist today, they are not as widespread as Buddhism or Yoga.

BUDDHISM
600–500 BCE

Siddhartha Gautama, later known as Buddha, leaves his privileged life to attain enlightenment and is believed to have learnt meditation from the Yogis. Gautama later diverges from this tradition and creates his own methodology to overcome suffering and move closer to enlightenment. This becomes Buddhism. Buddhist styles of meditation including Vipassana, Samatha, and Loving-Kindness, are some of the most widely practised forms of meditation in the West today.

 ## GREEK PHILOSOPHY
20 BCE–300 CE

Philosophers Philo of Alexandria and Plotinus develop meditation techniques involving concentration, but they are not embraced by early Christianity. The influence of Eastern thought and contemplative traditions in the West ends with the rise of Christianity in Europe.

| 500 BCE | 400 BCE | 200 BCE | 20 BCE |

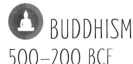 ## BUDDHISM
500–200 BCE

Buddhism spreads all over Asia, developing into many different lineages.

 ## GREEK PHILOSOPHY
327–325 BCE

Alexander the Great's military exploits in India are believed to have brought the Sages and Yogis of India in contact with the Greek philosophers. The Greeks develop their own forms of meditation, such as navel-gazing (*omphaloskepsis*).

CONTINUED ▶

UNDERSTANDING MEDITATION

18

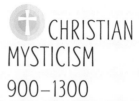

ZEN BUDDHISM
C.527

Bodhidharma, a Buddhist monk, is thought to have travelled from India to China to teach meditation, where he founds the Zen school of Buddhism. His teachings develop into the lineage of Chan in China, later spreading into Korea (Seon), Vietnam (Thien), and Japan (Zen), each of which practise variations of Zazen. Zazen is widely practised today.

CHRISTIAN MYSTICISM
500–600

The meditative practice of Lectio Divina features in The Rule of St. Benedict and is widely practised by Benedictine monks.

CHRISTIAN MYSTICISM
900–1300

Jesus Prayer is developed in Greece, in the Hesychasm Christian tradition. It is thought that this group of Christians was influenced by the Sufis or Indians.

300   500   600   900   1200

CHRISTIAN MYSTICISM
C.300

Christian Mystics develop their own form of meditation, mostly based on the repetition of a religious word or phrase, and the silent contemplation of God.

SUFISM
C.600S

Sufism, the mystical branch of Islam, is believed to have begun in the early period of Islam. The Sufis develop practices based on breathing, mantra, and gazing under some influence of Indian contemplative traditions. The core of their practice is to connect with God (Allah). The iconic Sufi Whirling (Samazen) is a form of dynamic meditation that can still be seen in Turkey.

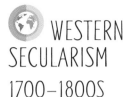

WESTERN SECULARISM
1893

Hindu missionary Swami Vivekananda attends and presents at the World Parliament of Religions in Chicago, triggering significant interest in Yoga and meditation in the West.

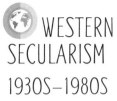

WESTERN SECULARISM
1900S

Several spiritual teachers migrate to the USA, including Paramahansa Yogananda, Maharishi Mahesh Yogi, and Swami Rama from India, and representatives of several schools of Buddhism. Meditation begins to be taught in a Westernized way, often simplified and decoupled from its spiritual context.

SIKHISM
1400S

Guru Nanak founds Sikhism in India. Sikh meditations, such as Kirtan, seek to feel God's presence. The tradition still exists among the Sikh community today.

WESTERN SECULARISM
1700–1800S

Several texts of Eastern philosophy are translated into European languages, including the *Upanishads* and *Bhagavad Gita*. The study of Buddhism in the West becomes a topic for intellectuals.

WESTERN SECULARISM
1930S–1980S

Scientific research about meditation begins to emerge, and it continues to move further away from its spiritual origins. As the number of studies about meditation increases, their quality also improves.

1300   1400   1700   1800   1900   1930   1980   TODAY

JEWISH KABBALAH
1200S

The Jewish mystical tradition of Kabbalah, originally an oral tradition, is collected in a group of texts called the Zohar. Several contemplatives develop meditation techniques in this tradition. They are largely based on the deep contemplation of philosophical principles, names of God, and the Tree of Life.

TODAY

Meditation is mainstream and is widely secularized. Its now proven benefits to the body, mind, and wellness are some of the most significant reasons for its continuing popularity.

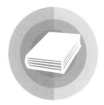

VEDANTIC

Abstract meditations that serve to contemplate who we truly are and free us from attachments.

NETI NETI. Rejecting all identification and attachment, and remaining as pure consciousness (pp.116–117).
SELF-ENQUIRY. Finding your real identity beyond all concepts, through the question "Who am I?" (pp.124–125).
WITNESSING. Focusing on the pure sense of "I am", and the fact that you are the conscious observer of all thoughts and sensations.

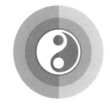

TAOIST

Practices that use the body, breath, and visualizations to empty yourself and find harmony with the Tao.

TAI CHI. Slow meditative movement (pp.96–97).
NEIGUAN. Inner visualization of the body (pp.98–99).
ZUOWANG (EMPTINESS MEDITATION). Letting all thoughts go and "forgetting about everything". Similar to Dzogchen (pp.126–127).
QIGONG. Breathing exercises with slow, synchronized body movement.

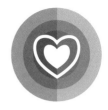

SUFI

Spiritual types of meditation from the mystics of Islam that have communion with God as their main goal.

HEARTBEAT MEDITATION. Focusing on the heart and listening to the heartbeat, or repeating mantras and thinking of God (pp.136–137).
ZIKR. Contemplating God (Allah) through the repetition of his sacred name, as in Mantra Meditation. Also called *muraqabah*.
BOND OF LOVE MEDITATION. Focusing on one's spiritual master.
SUFI WHIRLING/DANCE. Using music and body movement to achieve ecstatic states of union with the Beloved.

20

TAKING A CLOSER LOOK

Types of meditation

The practice of meditation goes back thousands of years, spanning many cultures and traditions (see pp.16–19), each with a variety of techniques. Here, we show the most significant types of meditation from the main traditions that are still widely practised. Some, such as Visualization, Third Eye, Abstract Meditation, Expand Your Consciousness, and Yoga Asanas, are common to more than one tradition or contain only some elements from them, so have not been included here.

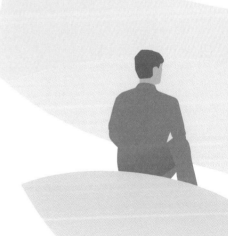

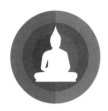

BUDDHIST AND ZEN

A broad spectrum of meditation practices that use concentration, observation, and pure awareness.

MINDFULNESS & VIPASSANA. Observing your present moment experience as it comes, without focusing on anything or attaching yourself to anything (pp.82–83 and pp.86–87).

ZAZEN. Concentrating on the breath, or on just sitting (pp.84–85).

KINHIN (ZEN WALKING MEDITATION). Walking slowly and focusing on your breath or on the sensations on the feet (pp.90–91).

LABELLING. Placing a label on every thought, feeling, and perception that arises (pp.112–113).

LOVING-KINDNESS. Kindling and growing the feeling of love for oneself and others (pp.134–135).

SAMATHA. Concentrating on the breathing, either through counting or through breathing sensations.

KOAN. Breaking through the conceptual mind using Zen riddles.

DZOGCHEN. A "do nothing" type of meditation, where attention neither focuses nor observes.

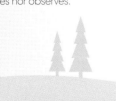

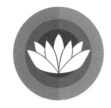

YOGIC

A variety of concentration-based practices that engage our sight, hearing, mind, heart, and energy.

PRANAYAMA. Regulated breathing techniques that alter your state of body and mind, such as Humming Bee Pranayama (pp. 88–89).

YOGA NIDRA. Practised lying down, it involves deep relaxation of all muscles, visualizations, and seeding a resolution or affirmation in the subconscious mind (pp.92–93).

KUNDALINI. Focusing the mind on the energy centres of the body (chakras). May include visualizations and the repetition of mantras (pp.100–101).

TRATAKA. Open-eye gazing meditation, usually on a candle flame, on a dot fixed on the wall, or on an image (pp.102–103).

MANDALA MEDITATION. Using geometrical images as an object of concentration (pp.106–107).

MANTRA MEDITATION. Repeating a word or phrase, silently or out loud (pp.110–111).

INNER SILENCE (ANTAR MOUNA). Observing the mind and senses, creating and disposing of thoughts at will, and then arriving at inner silence beyond all thoughts (pp.114–115).

TANTRIC MEDITATIONS, INCLUDING HEADLESS ME. Utilizing visualization, imagination, mantras, and sacred symbols to purify the mind and expand your consciousness (pp.128–133 and pp.120–121).

"The best technique is the one that works for you at this moment in your life."

SHARPENING YOUR POWERS

Meditation for your mind

Every time you meditate you sharpen your mental faculties, such as attention, awareness, and willpower. People have long recognized the psychological benefits of meditation, but recent research is able to show us how this works.

Let's say you start with the intention of focusing your attention on the breath and keeping it there for as long as possible. That is an exercise in attention and willpower. A few seconds later, you notice that your attention has wandered, and you're now thinking about what to have for lunch. That noticing itself is an exercise in self-awareness and mindfulness.

Then you disengage your attention from the thinking, and bring it back to your breathing. This is an exercise of mental flexibility (letting go), self-regulation, focus, and willpower. Your mind is being trained to be more fluid, to avoid rumination, and to be under your conscious control.

With time and continuous practice, these powers become sharper and sharper. In an age of technology and distraction, these are like superpowers.

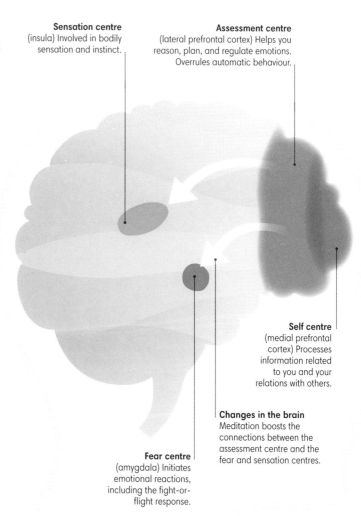

Sensation centre
(insula) Involved in bodily sensation and instinct.

Assessment centre
(lateral prefrontal cortex) Helps you reason, plan, and regulate emotions. Overrules automatic behaviour.

Self centre
(medial prefrontal cortex) Processes information related to you and your relations with others.

Changes in the brain
Meditation boosts the connections between the assessment centre and the fear and sensation centres.

Fear centre
(amygdala) Initiates emotional reactions, including the fight-or-flight response.

Rewiring the brain
Non-meditators have strong connections between the self centre and the fear and sensation centres. Meditation weakens these links and strengthens the pathways related to the assessment centre. The result is reduced anxiety and a tempered response to threats.

BRAIN BENEFITS

Research has proven that meditation has the following beneficial effects on our brains. The more you meditate, the stronger these changes in the brain become, so it's important to practise regularly. This maximizes the benefits and stops your brain slipping back to its default ways of working.

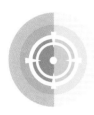

BETTER FOCUS

A 2010 US study found that participants' cognitive skills, including their ability to sustain attention and to perform under stress, was improved after meditating for just 20 minutes a day over four days. Meditation also boosted visuospatial processing, working memory, and executive functioning.

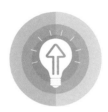

INCREASED CREATIVITY

A 2012 study by the University of Leiden assessed participants' creativity and "out-of-the-box" thinking by asking them to list alternate uses for common household items. Results showed that individuals performed better after open-monitoring meditation, which includes Mindfulness and Vipassana.

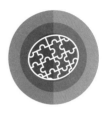

BETTER LEARNING AND MEMORY

After an eight-week mindfulness training programme, participants in a 2011 Harvard-affiliated study showed increased grey matter concentration in areas of the brain involved in learning and memory processes. They also showed an increase in areas related to taking perspective.

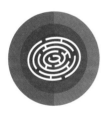

AWARENESS OF THE UNCONSCIOUS MIND

People who practise mindfulness meditation show more awareness of their intentions than those who do not meditate, according to research by the University of Sussex, England published in 2016. Meditators were also found to be harder to hypnotize.

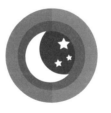

DECREASED NEED FOR SLEEP

A 2010 study by the University of Kentucky compared the normal sleep times of long-term meditators with non-meditators of the same age and gender. Results showed that the experienced meditators needed fewer hours of sleep.

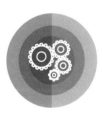

QUICKER PROCESSING

Research carried out in 2012 by scientists at the UCLA Laboratory of Neuro-Imaging found that long-term meditators have greater "gyrification" of the cortex than non-meditators, a phenomenon thought to help the brain process information and make decisions more quickly.

THE KEY TO EMOTIONAL WELLBEING

Meditation for your heart

By improving your skills of awareness, attention, and letting go, and with its many benefits to your health and mind, meditation can enhance your emotional and psychological wellbeing, laying the foundation for a happier, more balanced life.

Imagine you are going about your day, when someone cuts in front of you and the emotion of anger comes up. That feeling stresses your body and mind. In a way, it is a form of self-inflicted suffering.

Without meditation skills, that feeling may last for a long time. But with the skills of attention, awareness, and letting go that you learn through meditation, you can move on from that negative state much more quickly. Even while it is there, it doesn't occupy all of your awareness.

Some techniques, such as Loving-Kindness Meditation (see pp.134–135), also teach you how to purposefully cultivate positive emotions. The result is that you are able to spend less time and energy on negative emotions, and more on positive ones.

" *Negative emotions are no longer so deep and all-consuming.*"

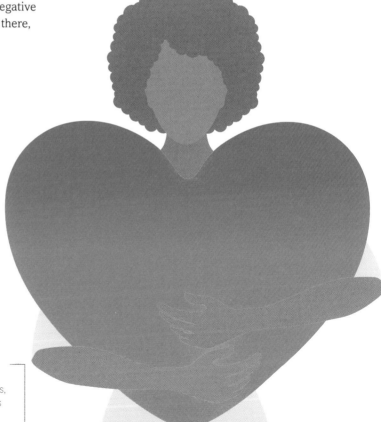

Love yourself
With its many benefits, meditation becomes a form of self-care.

WELLBEING BENEFITS

Research has shown that meditation has the following beneficial effects on our wellbeing. Many studies in this area focus on the Loving-Kindness technique, but benefits such as reduced depression and anxiety are common to several types of meditation.

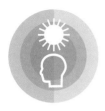

DECREASES DEPRESSION

A 2014 international study found that Mindfulness Meditation reduced symptoms of depression among adolescents compared with a control group. This was also found to be the case six months following the meditation training, suggesting that mindfulness also helps to prevent the development of depression-like symptoms.

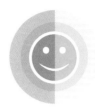

REGULATES ANXIETY AND MOOD DISORDERS

A 2006 study of 20 randomized controlled trials indicated that practising meditation has a positive effect on mood and anxiety disorders, while a US meta-analysis published in 2012 demonstrated that meditation techniques reduced symptoms of anxiety.

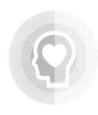

BOOSTS EMOTIONAL INTELLIGENCE AND RESILIENCE

Controlling your attention in meditation improves your resilience and emotional intelligence, according to psychotherapist Dr. Ron Alexander. Research from 2008 suggests that Loving-Kindness improves resilience in the face of change and adversity.

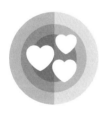

INCREASES EMPATHY

Practising a compassion-based meditation, such as Loving-Kindness, improves your ability to read the facial expressions of others, according to a US study published in 2013. The research also found that practitioners showed increased neural activity in areas of the brain related to empathy.

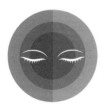

IMPROVES SELF-AWARENESS AND SELF-REGULATION

A US study published in 2011 showed that eight weeks of Mindfulness Meditation increased grey-matter concentration in areas of the brain related to regulating emotions, self-referential processing, and the ability to have perspective.

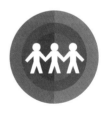

FOSTERS POSITIVE EMOTIONS AND HUMAN CONNECTION

Loving-Kindness Meditation boosted positive emotions among participants in a 2008 US study. This increased subjects' personal resources, such as purpose in life and social support. A US study from 2012 found that mindfulness decreased feelings of loneliness in older adults.

THE ZEN YOUR BODY NEEDS

Meditation and stress

Stress is a normal and necessary part of life, but too much stress can have a disastrous impact on our bodies. By giving you the tools to tackle stress both physically and emotionally, meditation helps you live a healthier life.

Whatever it stems from, stress is the feeling that you can't cope with what you're facing, and it can contribute to many health problems – from upsetting your digestive system and sleep, to encouraging unhealthy habits such as drinking too much alcohol and poor diet. In fact, it has been estimated that the majority of doctor's visits are stress-related.

By improving your skills of concentration, awareness, and relaxation, and your ability to choose what to focus on and manage your emotions (p.144),

meditation equips you to deal with stress in daily life, paving the way for a healthier mind and body. Meditation is also proven to reduce levels of the stress hormone cortisol, which is released as part of the fight-or-flight response. If the body's relaxation response doesn't get a chance to take effect before the next stressor, your cortisol levels remain elevated and you can enter a state of chronic stress, which has many negative outcomes for the body. Fortunately, meditation can break this cycle (see below).

Chronic stress leads to high levels of the hormone cortisol.

STRESS CYCLE

High levels of cortisol affect the functioning of the hippocampus, impairing your attention, perception, memory, and learning.

Poor performance leads to more stress, causing inadequate sleep and emotional distress, which also increase cortisol levels.

MEDITATION

All types of meditation help create a state of deep rest in your body and mind, which lowers cortisol levels and enables the hippocampus to function normally.

Breaking the stress cycle
Meditating regularly helps disrupt the chronic stress cycle so you can perform at your best.

STRESS BUSTING

As well as giving you the skills to tackle stress in your day-to-day life, meditation has been scientifically proven to reduce some of the physiological and psychological symptoms of stress.

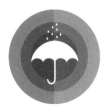

DECREASES REACTIVITY TO STRESS

Mindfulness has been found to be particularly good at decreasing our reactivity to stress, according to a 2015 British meta-analysis of research into meditation. As a result, we are able to experience stress in a more measured way.

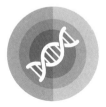

SLOWS AGEING

The shortening of telomeres, protective "caps" that stop DNA unravelling, has been linked to cellular ageing. By reducing stress arousal, some forms of meditation, such as Mindfulness, have a beneficial effect on telomere length, according to an American study published in 2009.

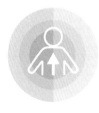

BOOSTS IMMUNITY

Stress can weaken the immune system, but meditation has been shown to counter this effect. A 2003 American study compared the immune response of meditators and non-meditators to a flu vaccine, and found that the meditators had greater immune function.

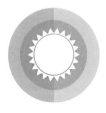

REDUCES SYMPTOMS OF PSYCHOLOGICAL STRESS

A 2014 American meta-analysis showed that Mindfulness Meditation programs decreased elements of stress, such as anxiety and pain. Another 2014 American meta-analysis found that the higher the level of anxiety participants reported, the greater the impact of meditation.

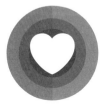

LOWERS BLOOD PRESSURE

High blood pressure is one of the many negative side-effects of stress, but a 2012 American study conducted between 1998 and 2007 found that blood pressure dropped among meditators. Meditators also had reduced risk of cardiovascular events, such as heart attacks.

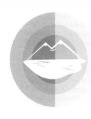

PROMOTES CALMNESS

Building meditation into your day can make you calmer. As part of a German study published in 2012, participants aged 18–65 who suffered from high levels of stress took part in a mindfulness-based walking program. The majority of participants reported feeling significantly calmer within four weeks.

THE ZEN YOUR BODY NEEDS

PRACTICAL SPIRITUALITY

Meditation for your soul

Spirituality was the original purpose of meditation, and its benefits, such as those shown here, can be significant. These often take longer to notice than the health and wellness benefits, but they meet a much deeper need.

"Peace is the foundation for existential happiness."

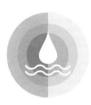

PURIFICATION OF MIND AND HEART

By shedding light on the unconscious mind, meditation enables you to free yourself from inner darkness.

MEDITATION MAKES US FACE OUR FEARS, our shadows, and ourselves. It brings to light everything we carry inside us, such as repressed memories, negative emotional patterns, and unexpressed feelings. In meditation, we bear witness to this psychological material, while keeping the mind calm and refraining from self-judgment and interpretations. Little by little, these thoughts and feelings are either released or integrated into our conscious mind and personality.

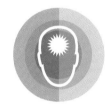

WISDOM, INSIGHT, AND ENLIGHTENMENT

Depending on how you approach your practice, meditation can involve a study of the deeper truths of life.

TRADITIONALLY, MEDITATION IS SEEN AS a way to cut through our illusions and reveal either the true nature of reality, as in the Buddhist and Taoist approaches, or our identity as the immortal Self, as in the Yogic and Vedantic approaches. The result is deeper insight into your "self", and greater wisdom about life. Along with the development of self-awareness, this can eventually lead to spiritual awakening or enlightenment, and the transcendence of suffering.

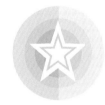

CONNECTION WITH "SOURCE"

For some, meditation is a time to connect with a higher power or reality – whatever that means to you.

MEDITATION IS A PAUSE IN YOUR LIFE when you don't engage with the exterior world. For some people, it is a time to connect to a higher reality, or power. This can help you experience a sense of oneness with other people and life in general, which soothes the pain of being an isolated individual and pushes you beyond the limits of your ego. Other forms of spiritual connection, such as prayer, chanting, contemplation, or selfless service, are enhanced by meditation practice.

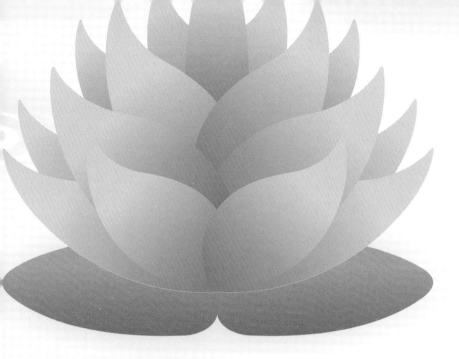

An ancient symbol
Revered in many cultures, the lotus represents purity and enlightenment.

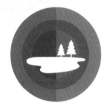

CONTENTMENT AND UNSHAKEABLE PEACE

As you begin to notice the benefits of meditation, you start to feel that everything will always be okay.

IT BECOMES OUR LIVED EXPERIENCE that, no matter how wrong things go, we are always able to access an inner shrine of stillness through meditation. This becomes the foundation for contentment with yourself and your life, and for happiness without a particular reason. Being happy for a reason is unsafe, because that reason may change. But if you are happy for no reason, if happiness or contentment is part of your being, then nobody can take that away from you.

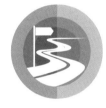

SENSE OF PURPOSE AND MEANING

Practised in a spiritual context, meditation is always part of a larger scheme or journey.

WHETHER MEDITATION SERVES to expand your human potential, connect with God, or achieve enlightenment, the result is the same: it gives a strong sense of purpose and meaning to your existence. As you try to align yourself with a higher power and make choices that help your spiritual growth, you no longer feel so lost in life. Otherwise, questions like "What is life for?" are never really tackled, and your material life, however successful, keeps failing to meet your deeper urges.

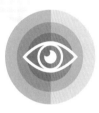

INCREASED INTUITION

Meditation helps us to give the thinking mind a break and tune in to something more powerful.

MANY OF US EXPERIENCE MOMENTS when we have direct knowledge of something without any apparent means to know it. Whether it is a flash of insight or a gut feeling, intuition can help us stay away from danger, understand the true motivations of people, and make difficult decisions in life. Meditation helps develop intuition by pausing our analytical mind. All techniques can improve this, but some, such as Trataka (see pp.102–103), are said to be more powerful.

A QUIET MIND

Turning the volume down

On average, we have about 50,000 thoughts a day, most of which we have already had many times. Awareness is the first step to quietening this mental chatter.

Suppose you wake up in the morning, go to the bathroom, and look at yourself in the mirror. It's most likely that your mind will mumble away, going on and on randomly, by itself, seemingly regardless of your will. Does that sound familiar? That is the default working mode of your mind.

MINDFUL THINKING

Thinking is what the mind does. There isn't much you can do about that. But with meditation, you can calm this noise down. Instead of being lost in your mental chatter, imagine going to the bathroom and washing your face while noticing the refreshing sensations of water touching your skin, brushing your teeth with a mindful focus on each tooth, and starting your day with more calmness and clarity. You recognize thoughts or monologues as they start to surface, and can choose to simply notice them and let them go, or play along with them, but with more purpose and awareness. This is what mindfulness feels like.

"...boring job..."

"...meeting with John today..."

"...need more sleep..."

"...I look terrible..."

"...it looks like it'll be a nice day..."

"....running late..."

Let it go
With more awareness, we can focus more on positive thoughts and let negative ones drift away, or be more present to the here and now.

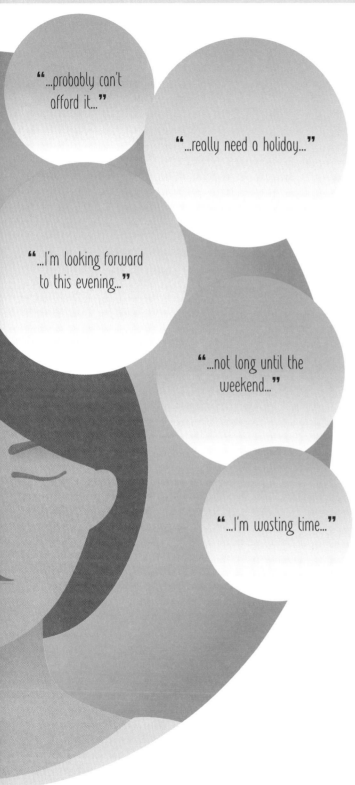

"...probably can't afford it..."

"...really need a holiday..."

"...I'm looking forward to this evening..."

"...not long until the weekend..."

"...I'm wasting time..."

BECOMING AWARE

The first step to quietening the noise in your mind is to develop the habit of watching your thoughts – a skill that you strengthen through meditation by becoming a witness to your mental and emotional states. With more awareness, you are able to distinguish the negative and unhelpful thoughts from the positive ones and can choose to let them go – just as you let go of distractions in meditation. As a result, your thoughts no longer ramble on and on by default and there is calm in your mind. This gives you space to decide where to focus your attention: whether that's whatever you are doing in the present moment, or a thought that is worth your attention, such as thinking about the next steps you need to take to achieve your goals.

"Awareness is the key to finding calm and peace in your mind."

YOU HAVE A CHOICE!

Mastering the flow

Are your thoughts always true? Are they even yours? We tend to believe our thoughts without question, but if we give them full authority, we can become their victim. Meditation teaches us that it's all about where we put our attention.

32

If your thoughts say "you are undeserving of love" or "you'll never amount to anything in life", then chances are that you will believe it, feel it, and act accordingly. But many of our thoughts are not true, or at least not helpful. They are a result of our memories, past conditioning, fears, and messages that we might have picked up from others. Even if we suspect that our thoughts are not always true, we may feel helpless in doing anything about it.

Instead, think of the flow of thoughts in your mind as a social media feed. Throughout your life you have "subscribed" to different things without even noticing. Now their posts keep showing up in your feed, and you don't know where they are coming from. Some are true and interesting, but many are depressing, unhelpful, or simply untrue.

THE POWER OF ATTENTION
Whether they're good or bad, helpful or unhelpful, attention feeds these thoughts. When you believe in a thought, identify with it, or develop an emotional reaction towards it, you make it stronger – just like sharing, liking, or commenting on a social media

post. But when you just observe it without involvement, it soon loses its energy and dissolves back into nothingness.

Meditation strengthens your powers of attention and focus by training you to constantly keep your attention on your meditation object. This enables you to redirect your attention away from unhelpful and untrue thoughts, and focus on feeding the good thoughts with your attention to make them stronger and to give them more power in your life (see opposite).

"You are not your thoughts, but simply the observer of them."

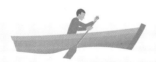

A MINDFUL MIND FLOW

The first step to mastering your mind flow is to be aware that you don't need to believe or follow your thoughts – this itself is an interruption to the mindless feed. Then, choose where to put your attention by asking two questions about each thought you have:

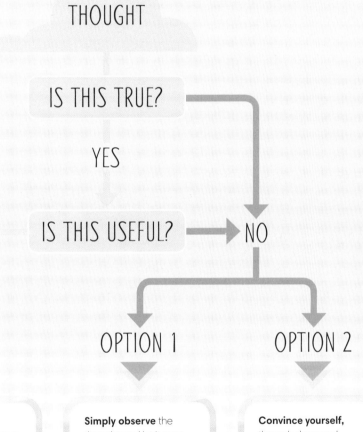

THOUGHT

IS THIS TRUE?

YES

IS THIS USEFUL? → **NO**

YES

OPTION 1

OPTION 2

Let the thought be.
You can like it, comment on it, expand it, share it, just like a social media post. Feel free to use it in your life, however you see fit. This will make the thought stronger.

Simply observe the thought and let it pass, without involvement, as you do in meditation. Your thought will go away eventually. It helps to put your attention somewhere else.

Convince yourself, through deep and mindful inner dialogue, exactly why the thought is not true or useful. This dialogue is particularly helpful for thoughts that recur frequently.

A HOUSE WITHOUT A MASTER IS CHAOS

The power of self-regulation

Without self-awareness, we are powerless in the face of our thoughts and feelings. Meditation gives us the tools to take back control of our mind and life.

34

Imagine a big house, with wonderful furniture, and plenty of food and sources of entertainment. There is only one problem: the house has no master. Since there is no master, anyone is allowed to come in, stay for as long as they like, and do whatever they want inside. Some people might make a lot of noise, break furniture, or bully the other guests, but nobody can do anything about it. There is a list of house rules, but because there is no master to enforce them, the rules are not respected. They are essentially just a wish list.

OUT OF CONTROL

Our mind is this chaotic house and the guests are all the thoughts, feelings, and emotions that visit it. The house rules are what we would like our life to be like – our values and aspirations – and the absent master is awareness. Without awareness, thoughts, feelings, and emotions are able to come in and create havoc in our minds. Nobody is watching over them, so they do

everything they can get away with. As a result, our mind becomes our greatest enemy, and we end up feeling far from who we want to be in life.

WAKING THE MASTER UP

All meditation practices are an exercise in awareness, attention, and self-regulation: they are essentially a wake-up call for the master of the house.

The more awareness you have about what is happening in your mind at all times, the more you will know yourself. Awareness is this quality of watchfulness, of presence. It looks inside and knows what is going on in your mind and heart. It can discern which guests should be allowed to stay and which ones should be shown the door before they do too much damage. Under the all-seeing eyes of awareness, you are able to regulate yourself and your life much better – the house rules are respected, and you once again feel like it's a good place to be.

YOUR HOUSE RULES

Your house rules, or values, represent what you want your inner life to be like. Deciding what they are will help you recognize which guests should be welcome, and which shouldn't be allowed to stay. Some examples could be:

BE POSITIVE and grateful.

LET GO of negative feelings.

LIVE IN the present moment.

DON'T RUN AWAY from your fears.

FOCUS ON what really matters.

"Be the master of your mind. Choose wisely where you place your attention."

LIVING IN THE MOMENT IS ONLY HALF THE STORY

Awareness in the present, past, and future

The message "be here now" is so often used in meditation that many people think present moment awareness is all there is to it. But developing our awareness through meditation can also be very helpful in thinking about our past and future.

Living in the moment, or present moment awareness, means that you are paying attention to what is happening right now. You are practising present moment awareness when you are eating and paying attention to the food you eat, or truly focusing while you are working, talking to someone, or exercising.

This type of awareness is a crucial element of meditation and there is no doubt that you need to be "here and now" in order to meditate, otherwise you will not realize when your mind has wandered during your practice. But although being "here and now" in your day-to-day activities brings a certain meditative quality to them, that by itself doesn't make them meditation – and it definitely doesn't replace the practice of a seated meditation. For true meditation, you also need relaxation, stillness, to look inside yourself, and to focus the mind (see pp.10–11).

A MINDFUL PAST AND FUTURE

Another common misconception is that thinking about the past or the future is somehow "against" the teachings of meditation. The ability to remember and learn from the past, to set goals, plan for the future, or think of the consequences of our actions, are all important skills for our everyday life. The problem happens when we become controlled and overwhelmed by the thoughts and feelings connected to our past and future – much like the house without a master (see pp.34–35).

Meditation practice doesn't ask you not to use these skills of memory, learning, or planning – nor does it reduce your ability to use them. In fact, the opposite is true: by teaching us to be aware of our thoughts, instead of this being a helpless habit over which we have no control, meditation helps us to engage with our past and future with more clarity, calmness, and purpose.

"Being present is an important part of meditation, but not the whole of it."

TRADITIONAL VS MEDITATIVE MINDSETS

By developing our awareness, meditation gives us the power to think consciously and deliberately, rather than automatically. With this comes a healthier relationship with our thoughts, the ability to put past and future in perspective, and to be more available to the present moment.

PAST

Thoughts and feelings about things you can't go back to – such as nostalgia or regrets – replay in your mind and can be overwhelming.

FUTURE

Thoughts and feelings about things yet to come – such as hopes and fears – take up space in your mind and cause anxiety.

AWARENESS

Your awareness is largely dominated by thoughts of the past and future.

PRESENT

You spend less time engaged in the present moment.

PAST

With more control over your attention, you can focus on the positives, such as lessons and memories.

AWARENESS

You have a calmer and clearer relationship with your thoughts about the past and future. You have more control over them and they occupy less space in your mind.

FUTURE

With more control over your attention, you can focus on the positives, such as your vision and goals.

PRESENT

You have more space in your mind to engage with the present moment and spend more time "in the now".

MEET THE MEDITATING MIND

STARTING YOUR JOURNEY

What to expect

In this chapter, you'll dive straight into some short meditations to give you a feel for different styles and bring some immediate calm to your life. But before you do, it can help to know what to expect.

First, dip your toe in the waters of meditation with a short, simple technique, then try each of the five mini-meditations at your own pace. Each mini-meditation has a different focus – the body, sight, breath, thought, and sound – which will give you a taste for the different techniques that are explored more fully in chapter 4. You may want to try the mini-meditations one after the other, but it is best to take your time so that you can really get a sense of how each one affects your body and mind, perhaps by spending 5 minutes a day trying one of them. You can also come back to and use these techniques any time you want to take a quick pause.

    Finally, you'll be prompted to reflect on how you felt before and after each meditation so that you can get a sense of which style works best for you, and to troubleshoot any immediate issues before you start setting up your daily practice.

REALISTIC EXPECTATIONS

With all that you have read about meditation in chapter 1, you might think that you'll become a superhuman after your first 10-minute session, but that's a trap. The benefits of meditation can take a while to show up – some may happen after a couple of weeks, while others may take months or even years. So if you go into your practice

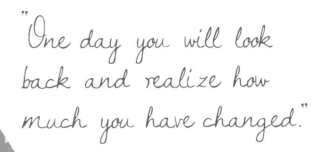

"One day you will look back and realize how much you have changed."

calculating the benefits and expecting immediate results, you are likely to feel disappointed and demotivated.

Having said that, depending on your sensitivity and level of self-awareness, there are some benefits that you may feel even after a single practice, such as:

- **Physical and mental** calmness and relaxation
- **Greater** mental clarity
- **Sense of freshness** and restfulness
- **Feeling grounded** and centered

As long as you follow the instructions as closely as you can, with the right mindset (see below), the benefits will come.

MEDITATOR'S MINDSET

The best attitudes to have regarding your practice are:

CURIOSITY. Develop a sense of openness and interest towards your practice so it doesn't become mechanical or boring.

PERSEVERANCE. Commit to meditating every day, no matter what. This is the foundation of all the benefits and transformations that meditation can bring (p.62).

NO-JUDGMENT. Don't criticize or blame yourself for getting distracted during the practice, or for not doing it "right". Refrain from over-evaluating your sessions.

PATIENCE. Don't hurry and don't expect too much too soon. Self-transformation takes time.

TAKE A BREATH

Your first taste of meditation

If you've never meditated before, or if you just want to take a pause before continuing with your meditation journey, try this short meditation. It will only take you 5 minutes – you can even put on a timer, if you like.

01 Sit down comfortably, in a chair or on the floor. Keep your back and neck straight. Either close your eyes or keep them open, but in a relaxed and still gaze, towards the floor.

02 Take three deep breaths in through your nose, and out through your mouth. Then close your mouth.

03 Ground yourself in your body. Your body is here and now. Feel the weight of your body. Feel the shape of your whole body. Feel the sensations of your body touching the floor, and your skin touching your clothes.

04 Mentally scan your body for any tensions. When you find one, focus on it, and have the feeling that you are releasing it as you exhale.

"At any stage in this process, if thoughts or images arise, just let them be. Don't feel disturbed by them."

05 Bring your attention to your breathing. Notice which parts of your body are involved in the breathing process: the nostrils, throat, chest, abdomen. Observe the sensations of breathing in all these parts of your body.

06 Pay attention to the sensations of breathing in the nostrils. What is the quality of your breathing? Deep or shallow? Slow or fast? Even or jerky? Warm or cold?

07 Imagine that your thoughts are passing by like clouds in the sky, and keep observing your breath sensations.

08 Ask yourself: "Compared to 5 minutes ago, what has changed in my body and mind?" Try to feel the difference.

NOW TRY MINI-MEDITATION 1

Grounded as a Mountain
Use body awareness and affirmations to feel still and solid ▶

GROUNDED AS A MOUNTAIN

Mini-meditation 1: body awareness

A mountain is a symbol of peace, strength, and power. Using your imagination, affirmations, and body awareness, this meditation makes you feel as still and stable as a mountain. It can also be used before any other meditation, or to help you fall asleep.

01 Sit in a stable and comfortable posture. Close your eyes, then take three deep breaths through your nose. Make them long, soft, and even.

02 Take a few moments to feel your entire body as a single unit. Feel the contact of your body with the floor, cushion, or chair. Feel how the ground supports you.

03 Bring your focused awareness to your whole right leg, from buttock to toes. Repeat to yourself:

04 As you say these words, imagine your leg becoming a mountain. It's as if a mountain is growing from within your body, or your cells are turning the "mountain mode" on.

"...My right leg is as heavy as a mountain. As solid as a mountain. Fully relaxed, comfortable, and still.**"**

06 Focus on your whole body again, as a single unit. Notice how it feels. Repeat to yourself:

"...My whole body is as heavy as a mountain. As solid as a mountain. Fully relaxed, comfortable, and still.**"**

07 Feel how restful, peaceful, and pleasurable it is to experience that deep sense of physical stillness. Enjoy the sense of relaxation and sinking in.

05 Repeat the same affirmations for the other areas of your body: your left leg (from buttock to toes), each arm (shoulder to fingertips), then torso, neck, head, and face.

08 Whenever you're ready, bring your attention to your fingers and start slowly moving them. Then, body part by body part, slowly come out of the meditation.

09 When you've finished, take a few moments to reflect on how you felt during and after (see pp.54–55).

"Say the words with conviction, focus, and feeling. Awaken these feelings in your body."

NOW TRY MINI-MEDITATION 2

Steady Gazing
The next meditation uses the stillness of the eyes to still the mind ▶

STEADY GAZING

Mini-meditation 2: stilling the mind

By keeping your gaze still, this technique creates stillness in the mind. Trataka (see pp.102–103) is a more elaborate version, but this variation is really simple. It can also be used as a preparation for any other meditation.

01 Sit or lie down in a stable and comfortable posture. Keep your eyes open and take three deep breaths through your nose. Make them long, soft, and even. Relax your body and keep it stable throughout the meditation.

02 Find an unmoving object to focus on, such as a building, the moon, or an object on your desk. Move your body and head in that direction. Ideally, have the object at eye level, so your head and eyes are parallel with the floor. If the object is large, choose one part to focus on.

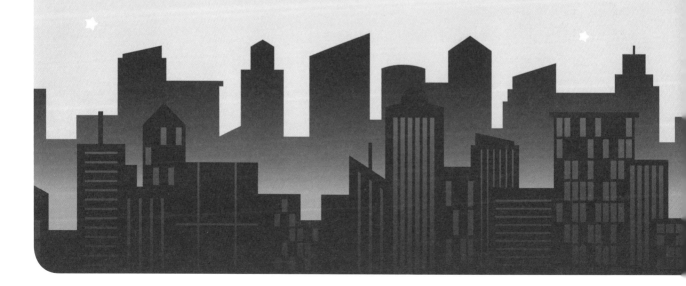

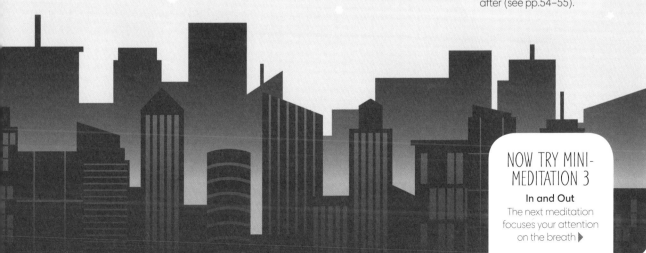

"Have your whole awareness become one with your eyes."

03 Fix your eyes and mind on your object, as if it is the only thing that exists in the entire universe. Keep your eyes still but relaxed. Don't blink intentionally, but let it happen naturally. If you are frowning or your eyes are flickering, you are tensing too much. You also shouldn't feel any burning in the eyes. If you do, stop the practice.

04 Let thoughts come and go like clouds in the sky. If you find it helpful, repeat the name of the object in your mind as a mantra, for example "moon, moon, moon". This will help to centre your thoughts on the object, together with your gaze. Continue for 3–5 minutes.

05 When you are ready, close your eyes and rest them a little. Then, take a few moments to reflect on how you felt during and after (see pp.54–55).

STEADY GAZING

NOW TRY MINI-MEDITATION 3
In and Out
The next meditation focuses your attention on the breath ▶

IN AND OUT

Mini-meditation 3: counting your breaths

The breath is one of the most popular meditation objects. You can pay attention to breathing sensations, sync your breath with a mantra, or modulate it in specific patterns. This technique follows the easiest method: counting your breaths.

01 Sit or lie down in a stable and comfortable posture. Take three deep breaths in through your nose and out through your mouth. Make them long, soft, and even. Relax your body and keep it stable throughout the meditation. Close your eyes and mouth.

02 Bring your attention to your breath. Observe its flow for a few moments. Don't try to change it – simply observe it as it is.

03 Now start counting your breaths from 10 to 1. Breathe in and, at the end of your inhalation, mentally say the number "10". Then breathe out. At the end of your exhalation, mentally count "10" again. Then repeat for 9-9, 8-8, all the way down to 1. When you arrive at 1, start another cycle from 10.

06 Spend a few moments reflecting on how you felt during and after the meditation (see pp.54–55).

05 When you feel ready, stop counting and observe your breathing for a few moments. Notice any changes in your breathing pattern and in your mind. Gently move your fingers, open your eyes, and conclude the practice.

04 As you count, let thoughts come and go – there is no need to suppress them or to be bothered by them. Just make sure that you allocate enough attention to your breathing and counting so you don't lose track.

"If you get lost or forget the last number, start again from 10."

NOW TRY MINI-MEDITATION 4
Clouds in the Sky
Use "observing awareness" to gain calm and clarity ▶

CLOUDS IN THE SKY

Mini-meditation 4: observing your thoughts

By default, we consider our thoughts to be facts. We may even have a strong identification with them (see pp.32–33). In this meditation you become a witness to your thoughts, which helps you get some distance from them and gives you greater clarity and inner freedom.

02 Imagine "taking a step back" inside your mind, and watching your thoughts pass by like clouds in the sky. Each cloud has a different shape, colour, speed, and meaning, but they are all still just clouds, and they are all passing by. Observe them from a distance.

01 Sit or lie down in a stable and comfortable posture. Take three deep breaths in through your nose and out through your mouth. Make them long, soft, and even. Relax your body and keep it stable throughout the practice.

"When you notice that your attention has been drawn to a thought, simply bring your mind back to pure observing."

"Your thoughts may be words, feelings, or images, but think of them all as clouds."

03 Allow yourself to notice each thought, but do not interact with it. Don't interpret the thought, don't judge it, and don't have any dialogue with it. Remain the impartial observer of every thought that arises. That's all you need to do. Practise this for a few minutes.

04 When you're ready, slowly start moving your body, then open your eyes. Take a few moments to reflect on how you felt during and after (see pp.54–55).

YOUR OBSERVER MINDSET

If the image of clouds doesn't work for you, you can try different visual metaphors:

YOUR THOUGHTS ARE LIKE BUBBLES in a creek – you are watching them pass by.

YOUR THOUGHTS ARE LIKE IMAGES projected on a cinema screen – you are watching them play like a film.

NOW TRY MINI-MEDITATION 5

The Sound of Now
Focus on the sense of hearing to empty the mind ▶

THE SOUND OF NOW

Mini-meditation 5: pure receptivity

This meditation uses your sense of hearing to achieve a state of pure receptivity. Your ears cannot think, so the more you focus all your awareness on simply hearing, the more you empty your mind of everything else, creating space, peace, and clarity.

01 Sit or lie down in a stable and comfortable posture. Take three deep breaths in through your nose and out through your mouth. Make them long, soft, and even. Then close your mouth. Relax your body and keep it stable throughout the practice.

02 Bring all your awareness to your sense of hearing. Imagine that it is your only sense, your only way of perceiving the world. Let your whole mind become your ears.

03 Scan your environment for sounds. Notice as many as you can – it could be birdsong, the dishwasher, or cars passing in the background. You don't need to name them in your mind, or think about where they are coming from. Don't get stuck on any one sound, just spend a few seconds on each.

"If any thoughts or other sensations distract you, bring your attention back to pure listening."

04 Gradually move your hearing to more distant sounds, away from your body. Experience every sound as it is, without likes or dislikes. It's just pure listening, as if you were a rock with ears.

07 When you are ready, let go of your sound and bring your attention back to your body. Notice how you feel. Gently move your fingers, open your eyes, and finish the practice. Take a moment to reflect (see pp.54–55).

05 Now choose one sound that you can hear continuously in your environment. If you can't find anything that is constant, pay attention to the sound of your breathing.

06 Your goal is not to block all other sounds from your mind, but simply to keep an unbroken stream of awareness on the sound you choose.

NOW IT'S TIME TO REFLECT

How did that feel?
Take a pause to think about how you felt in each meditation ▶

HOW DID THAT FEEL?

Time to reflect

Now that you've tried meditation for yourself, take some time to think about how it made you feel. You may already be feeling calm and peaceful but, as with learning any new skill, it can take time. If you're experiencing any issues, it's likely they have simple solutions.

Q WHAT SHOULD I DO NEXT?

Each of the mini-meditations (see pp.44–53) has a different focus – body, sight, breath, thoughts, and sound. Reflecting on how each technique made you feel will help you get a sense of which type of meditation might work for you as your build your practice. Ask yourself the following questions about each mini-meditation:

● **How did you feel during** the meditation? Was your mind naturally engaged with the practice and at ease, or did you find it boring and forceful? Different sensory channels have a stronger appeal for different people, so consider which sensory focus worked best for you, and choose a technique that works primarily on that one.

● **How did you feel after** each meditation? People meditate for different purposes, experiences, or personal developments. You may just want to relax, or you may want to experience a sense of freedom, presence, love, or self-knowledge. Think about what you seek most, and which of the mini-meditations helped you to achieve that, then choose a similar technique in chapter 4 to try next.

Q THIS FEELS ODD – AM I DOING IT RIGHT?

You may feel a sense of peace and rest from your first meditation, or perhaps just a basic relaxation. Others may experience things that they find hard to articulate or understand. You may also feel unsure about whether you are following the instructions correctly, for example, if you struggled to create the feeling of relaxation and heaviness in your body (see pp.44–45), or were unsure about the difference between thinking and observing thoughts (see pp.50–51). Whatever you feel, it is best not to worry about it at this point. As you continue to practise and learn about meditation, things will become clearer.

Q HOW CAN I STOP FALLING ASLEEP WHEN I MEDITATE?

This a very common problem. Firstly, make sure you are getting enough sleep, otherwise you will feel sleepy and frustrated during your meditation. Then, check that you are meditating at an optimal time of day (see p.58).

The final point is posture. If you can, meditate upright, with your back straight and unsupported. This helps to keep the mind alert. If you need to meditate lying down, raise your knees and place the soles of your feet flat on the floor (see p.68).

If you are still struggling to stay awake, try shortening your sessions and increasing them gradually. With time, your mind will learn to be calm and alert without reverting to sleep.

Q HOW CAN I MAKE MY MIND LESS RESTLESS?

It can feel like our attention has a mind of its own: it goes after what it likes and stays there as long as it likes, no matter what you want it to do.

Meditation is not about fighting with the mind, rejecting thoughts, or suppressing anything – it's about training your awareness and focus. Let the

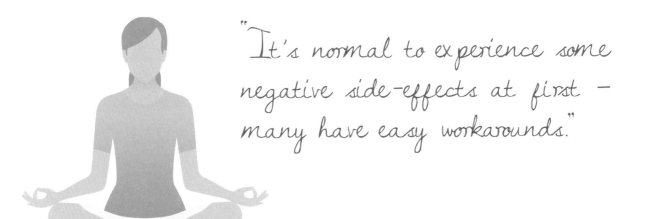

"It's normal to experience some negative side-effects at first – many have easy workarounds."

mind be as it is, but make the effort of putting your attention into the practice. To begin with, this is about noticing distractions as often and as quickly as you can. Every time you notice that your mind has wandered, you strengthen your awareness muscle. That is good – feel happy about it! Do your best and accept the results.

It also helps to understand how attention works. Our attention will always naturally go towards an object that is related to our likes, dislikes, or identity. We can't change this tendency, but we can use it in our favour. First, make sure you choose a meditation that you naturally enjoy. Then, learn to enjoy your meditation object. If you choose a technique that focuses on the breath, for example, try to develop a sense of enjoyment around it – feel that each breath is deeply interesting, mysterious, and pleasurable.

Q SHOULD MEDITATION HURT MY BACK, KNEES, OR LEGS?

Meditation doesn't need to be painful. Make sure that you follow the posture guidelines, or try a lying-down position (see pp.66–69).

Q WHAT SHOULD I DO IF MY BODY ITCHES DURING MEDITATION?

Practising a full body scan and relaxation (see pp.44–45 or pp.92–93) for a few minutes before your main practice should decrease any urge you have to itch. If you still feel an itch, try to simply watch that urge: take a mindful pause and relax that sensation. If you still absolutely need to itch, do it slowly and get back to your meditation.

Q IS IT NORMAL FOR MY BREATH TO BECOME RESTLESS AND UNNATURAL WHEN I'M WATCHING IT?

This can happen. Simply accept that the breathing pattern will be like this for a while. Don't judge yourself, don't tense up, and don't panic: relax and let the breathing be as it is. It will normalize with time and practice.

Q I'M STILL EXPERIENCING DIFFICULTIES – WHAT DO I DO?

Most side-effects will pass after a few sessions. If they do continue for a while, try changing your technique, or consult a meditation teacher.

STARTING
YOUR PRACTICE

SETTING UP A DAILY PRACTICE

Why, when, how long, where, and how

Any amount of meditation is better than no meditation at all, but to get the most out of your practice you need to meditate every day. Establishing a practice that works well for you will help make meditation a daily habit.

The more closely you can follow these guidelines, the easier it will be for you to settle into and deepen your practice, but don't let your current situation be an excuse for you not to practise: start from where you are and do what you can.

WHY?

Firstly, it helps to be clear on the reasons why you want to meditate. Is it for the health benefits? Stress relief? Increased performance? Wellbeing? Emotional healing? Spiritual growth and connection? Make a list of the main things that motivate you to meditate and refer to it when you are lacking motivation. It may help to consider the many benefits of meditation described in chapter 1.

The more clarity you have about why you want to meditate, the stronger your motivation to practise will be. This will be the fuel for your daily meditation session and will determine how far you will go in it.

WHEN?

It is best to always meditate around the same time every day as this helps establish it as a habit. Many people meditate in the morning because it is easier to make sure you don't skip it, but you can choose a time of day that works for you, according to your routine, as long as it follows the guidelines shown here. Ideally, pick a time when you feel rested, refreshed, and alert, otherwise it will be very hard to go deep in your practice. This means it is good to meditate:

● **In the morning,** after a good night of sleep, so you feel well rested.
● **A few minutes after** light exercise, provided you let your body settle, as you are likely to be more alert.
● **Any time when** your stomach is empty (at least 2 hours after a large meal), as digesting food can make you feel sleepy.

Your body clock
Meditating at the same time every day helps your body and mind know when to settle and focus.

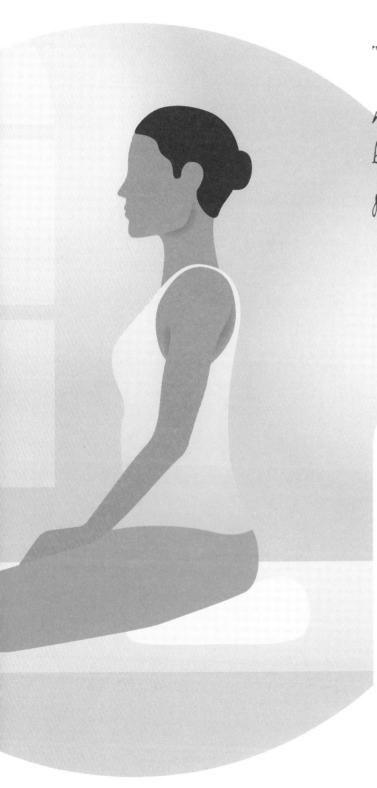

"With time,
meditation will
become just another
part of your day."

GETTING INTO GOOD HABITS

To establish any new habit, it helps to perform it directly after another habitual action, known as an anchor habit. For meditation, this will need to be something that you do every day, around the time you'd like to meditate.

IF YOU WANT TO MEDITATE in the morning, for example, your anchor habit could be taking a shower. This means that in your mind you associate meditation with the next thing to do after showering. Other examples of anchor habits could be having a glass of water in the morning, or brushing your teeth. It can be anything, as long as it happens on a daily basis.

YOU'LL THEN NEED TO CHOOSE a trigger that will remind you to meditate. This will only be needed for the first few weeks, when your habit is still not established. A trigger could be a sticky note on your mirror or an alarm on your phone.

CONTINUED ▶

HOW LONG?

Start with short sessions so you don't risk overstretching your motivation and so you have no excuse to skip it – even a 5-minute session is enough in the beginning. As time passes, if your habit is established and you are enjoying your practice, you can gradually increase the length, for example, by 1 minute a week. For the general benefits of meditation, you should ultimately aim for your daily sessions to last for 20 minutes. For deeper self-transformation or spiritual benefits, aim for 40 minutes. You can use a timer or a meditation app to measure your sessions.

WHERE?

Think of somewhere quiet in your home or workplace where you will ideally not be disturbed. Privacy is also crucial so you feel safe to close your eyes and look inside yourself.

Our environment impacts our mind so, if you can, choose a place free from distractions, uncluttered, tidy, and clean. Most people find it impractical to have a space entirely dedicated to meditation, so identify even just a corner of a room where you will always practise.

It's important to try to meditate in the same place every day, when you can. This helps to build a strong habit and creates associations that will enable you to ease into the practice when you enter that space. The space becomes a trigger for the mind to calm down and relax.

You can also bring meditation into other areas of life, such as at work, on your commute, while walking, or just sitting in a park (see pp.140–141).

HOW?

Many techniques are taught in this book, so choose a few that you wish to experiment with (see pp.80–81) or, if you already know the technique you like the most, stick to that one.

It's also a good idea to choose your sitting position – either on the floor, a bench, or a chair (see pp.66–69) – and arrange any props that you may need, such as a candle or mandala. Leave them in your meditation place so you can easily access them when it's time to meditate.

RINSE AND REPEAT

At the end of every practice, regardless of the quality of that meditation, take a moment to appreciate that you took the time to do something good for yourself, something important. Then recommit to meditating again the following day, in the same time and place.

Finally, throughout your practice, keep the "meditator's mind-set" of curiosity, perseverance, no-judgment, and patience in relation to your practice (see pp.40–41).

"Building meditation into your day will help you advance in your practice."

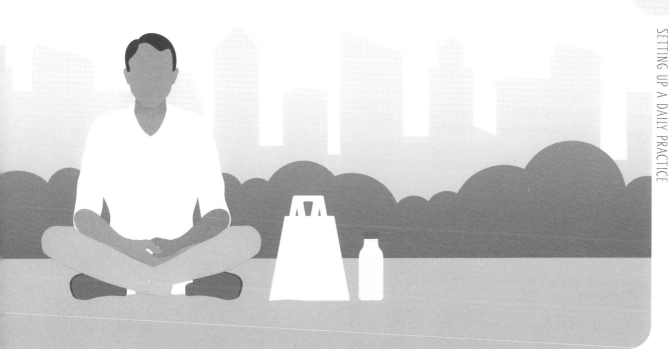

61

NEVER ZERO

The power of commitment

No matter how motivated you are, developing any new habit can be difficult. Motivation is the initial fuel you need to get going, but it can be as volatile as your mood. Once you've started, you'll need commitment to make meditation part of your life for the long term.

It is commitment that keeps a married couple going, despite moments of conflict and difficult times. It is commitment that makes a burnt-out parent continue to strive to provide the best for their children. And it is commitment that will keep you meditating, even when you are feeling tired, busy, or demotivated.

In building a meditation habit, this commitment has a name: never zero. Never zero means that you tell yourself: "I will meditate every day. I won't go to sleep without meditating, come what may! Even if I am tired, even if I am super busy, even if I am travelling, I'll make the time to sit for at least 5 minutes." The moment you make this sincere commitment to yourself, meditation starts to take deep roots in your life. It means you have already won the first battle: that of discipline.

THE FREEDOM OF COMMITMENT

The never zero commitment frees up a lot of mental space: it means that you will never again need to decide if you will meditate today or not, or if you have time for it or not. If circumstances are particularly challenging in a given day, your only question needs to be: "When can I meditate today? And for how long?"

If you're not ready to make this commitment to yourself just yet, that's okay. You can still explore meditation, learn more about it, and try it out. But it is only once you make this commitment that you will be able to access all the benefits that meditation can bring for you.

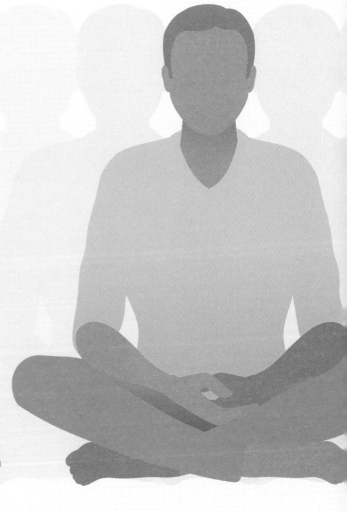

"There is tremendous power in doing something positive for yourself every day, no matter what."

EXCUSES, EXCUSES

Have it clear in your mind that "never zero" doesn't accept any exceptions. Spend a minute thinking of all the challenging circumstances that may come up, and that give you the perfect excuse to skip or "forget" your practice that day. Then, think of a counter-argument. For example:

EXCUSES

"I have a big deadline coming up and work is my priority — I'll catch up tomorrow."

"I can't meditate in my usual place or time today, so that means I can't meditate."

"I'm on holiday, so that means I can take a break from meditation too."

"I have too much going on emotionally at the moment — I can't face meditating."

AFFIRMATIONS

"Meditation helps me perform at my best. It's a good use of my time."

"This is a great opportunity to practise bringing meditation into my daily life."

"Meditation makes me feel relaxed and calm. It will help get the most out of my break."

"I am just a witness to difficult thoughts. Meditation helps me process them."

ENJOY THE PROCESS

The foundation for lifelong practice

The more you enjoy meditation, the more you will get out of your practice. If you cultivate positivity around it, you are also more likely to stay motivated and committed to your meditative journey, creating the foundation for it to become a long-term habit.

Learning to enjoy the process is all about your relationship with meditation, and the inner dialogue that you have about your practice. The key is to remember that meditation is a special time that you set aside for yourself, rather than a task to cross off your to-do list. It is about getting to know yourself, befriending yourself, and mastering yourself, and is a force multiplier for everything else in life.

Try any of the following ideas to help keep meditation an enjoyable part of your life.

● **See meditation as a journey** of exploration. Think about your practice, explore different methods, and meet different teachers, until you find what works best for you.

● **Make sure you are meditating in the best conditions,** such as creating an inspiring place to meditate and using a good cushion or stool (see p.60 and pp.66–69).

● **Try not to develop negative feelings** around your practice, such as criticizing yourself or over-analyzing your sessions. Understand that just showing up and exercising your awareness and focus skills is all you need to do (see right).

● **Meditate just a little less** than you would like to. Don't stretch your motivation – this helps to keep the hunger alive.

● **Find a meditation partner** – someone that is enthusiastic about the practice and with whom you can exchange experiences.

● **Join a friendly meditation community** to keep you inspired and on track.

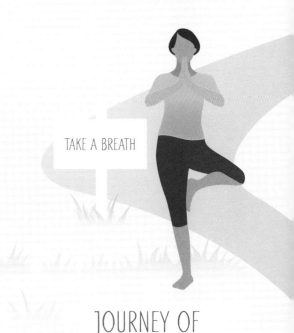

TAKE A BREATH

JOURNEY OF EXPLORATION

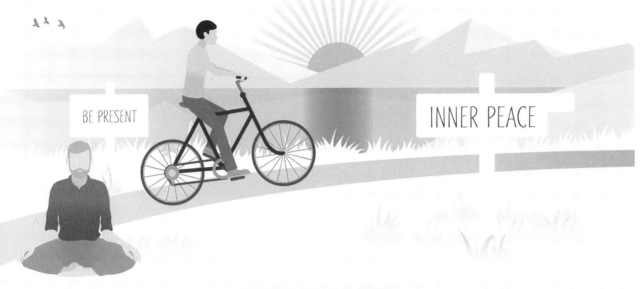

INNER DIALOGUE

If you find yourself slipping into negative self-talk, counter that thought with a positive one, as in the examples below. Notice how the negative ways of thinking close you down, while the positive ones uplift you, encourage you, and open you up.

NEGATIVE SELF-TALK

"I need to get my meditation done so I can get on with my day."

"Meditation is boring, but I do it because I know it's good for me."

"I have to meditate. It's a necessary chore."

"Everyone meditates, everyone knows meditation is good for you. I would feel ashamed if I didn't do it."

POSITIVE SELF-TALK

"Great, it's time to treat myself to some Zen!"

"I love how I feel after a good meditation. It's so nourishing and refreshing!"

"Meditation is an exploration into the depths of my being."

"I experience a unique sense of peace and wellbeing through meditation, and I want more of that."

65

ENJOY THE PROCESS

AN EMPOWERED POSTURE

Establishing a strong foundation

Slouching on a sofa makes you feel tired or lethargic, while standing up tall makes you feel confident and strong. Your body influences your mind, so finding the right meditation posture is crucial for your practice.

Body language is a powerful tool in telling your nervous system how you should be feeling, so it's important to follow specific recommendations for the meditation postures. These postures are not part of a ritual, or a cultural symbol, but the result of centuries of experiments into how certain positions affect the mind. As long as you follow the guidelines on these pages, you will develop a strong foundation for your practice.

CHOOSING A POSE

These pages show four postures that you can use in meditation. It is best to meditate on a cushion on the floor (see right), as this is the most stable meditation posture, making it easier for you to relax and achieve physical and mental stillness. Sitting on a cushion will feel more natural with practice, but if you find it too difficult, you can apply the same principles to meditating on a stool or chair to get the right balance of comfort and stability. You can also meditate lying down if sitting upright is too uncomfortable (see pp.68–69).

" A good posture is the best foundation for meditative practice."

04 To help keep your neck straight, gently lift the top of your head towards the ceiling, as if it is being pulled by an invisible string.

03 Close your eyes and mouth.

02 Keep your spine and neck straight, without leaning on anything.

01 Tilt the upper part of your pelvis forward slightly – this will help keep your back straight more effortlessly.

THE BURMESE POSITION

To adopt the Burmese position, shown here, you can sit on a cushion, folded blanket, or yoga block, as long as your hips are just higher than your knees. With time, your hips will become more flexible, making it easier to sit this way.

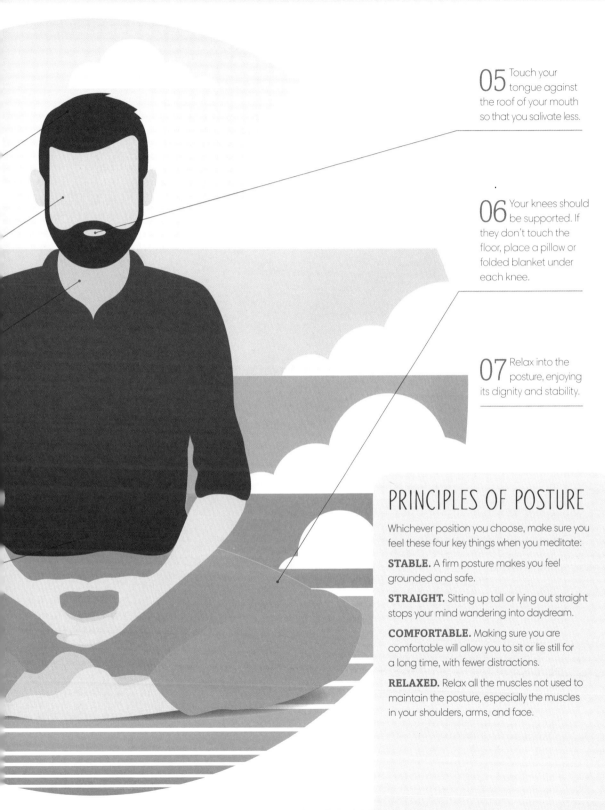

05 Touch your tongue against the roof of your mouth so that you salivate less.

06 Your knees should be supported. If they don't touch the floor, place a pillow or folded blanket under each knee.

07 Relax into the posture, enjoying its dignity and stability.

PRINCIPLES OF POSTURE

Whichever position you choose, make sure you feel these four key things when you meditate:

STABLE. A firm posture makes you feel grounded and safe.

STRAIGHT. Sitting up tall or lying out straight stops your mind wandering into daydream.

COMFORTABLE. Making sure you are comfortable will allow you to sit or lie still for a long time, with fewer distractions.

RELAXED. Relax all the muscles not used to maintain the posture, especially the muscles in your shoulders, arms, and face.

CONTINUED ▶

ALTERNATIVE POSTURES

If you find sitting cross-legged, as in the Burmese position, too uncomfortable, you can meditate on a stool, on a chair, or lying down. Whichever you choose, make sure that you are following the principles of posture (see p.67). Then, close your eyes and mouth, touch your tongue against the roof of your mouth, and relax.

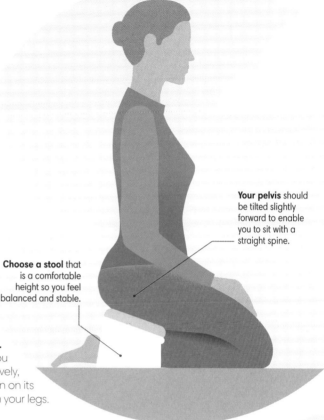

Your pelvis should be tilted slightly forward to enable you to sit with a straight spine.

Choose a stool that is a comfortable height so you feel balanced and stable.

MEDITATING ON A STOOL

To meditate in a kneeling position, you usually use a stool or bench. Alternatively, you can turn a meditation cushion on its side and place it between your legs.

"*If you meditate lying down, have a strong intention of not falling asleep.*"

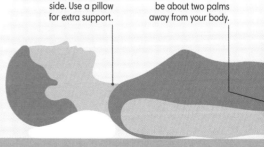

Tilt your head up to straighten your neck. Don't let your head fall to the side. Use a pillow for extra support.

Your hands should be about two palms away from your body.

MEDITATING LYING DOWN

If sitting causes great discomfort, meditate lying down. It can be challenging not to fall asleep, so you can try placing the soles of your feet flat on the floor – if you drift off, your legs will fall outwards, waking you up.

MEDITATING ON A CHAIR

If meditating on a cushion or a stool doesn't work for you, you can try meditating on a chair. Be sure to select a chair that is stable and allows you to sit up straight with your feet fully touching the ground. Even if your chair has a back support, it is best not to lean back.

Your thighs should be parallel to the floor.

You can use a cushion to tilt your pelvis forward slightly, which helps to keep your spine straight.

Your neck, head, and spine should form a straight line.

Surrender your whole body to the floor, letting go of all tensions.

Keep your hands open with palms facing up and fingers relaxed.

Keep your legs slightly wider than shoulder-width apart, allowing your feet to fall outwards.

"You can use the chair posture to meditate any time, anywhere."

A BREATH OF FRESH AIR

Abdominal breathing

Every cell in your body needs a constant influx of oxygen, so how you breathe has a deeper impact on your wellbeing than you might expect. Breathing abdominally helps you to relax in meditation and stay calm and composed in daily life.

Chest breathing only fills the middle areas of the lungs and causes strain to your shoulders and neck. It also activates the flight-or-fight mode in your body, increasing the stress hormone cortisol.

When you breathe abdominally, however, oxygen reaches the bottom part of your lungs where the blood vessels are most concentrated. As a result, your body gets more oxygen with less effort, helping improve your mood and raise your energy levels. It also has a calming effect on your body and mind, enabling you to achieve a greater state of relaxation during meditation, while breathing abdominally all the time will bring these benefits to the rest of your life. Ideally, you should also breathe through the nose, and keep the breath slow and deep.

HOW DO YOU BREATHE?

To find out what your default mode of breathing is, lie down and place your left hand on your belly, and your right on your chest. Breathe normally. If your left hand moves, you breathe through the abdomen. If your right hand moves, you breathe through your chest.

If you are a chronic chest breather, the exercise shown right will help you change your default breathing mode to abdominal. This might feel unnatural at first, but after a week of daily practice, it should feel much easier.

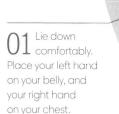

02 Spend 1 minute just observing the natural flow of breath and how it is moving your body and your hands. Don't attempt to change it yet.

01 Lie down comfortably. Place your left hand on your belly, and your right hand on your chest.

How to breathe abdominally
Do the following exercise every morning and evening for three weeks. Check in with your breath during the day and make a conscious shift if needed.

03 Focus your attention on your left hand and your abdomen. Continue breathing normally, but keep your focus there. Do this for 1 minute.

04 As you breathe in, allow your diaphragm to expand downward, causing your belly to move forward and slightly outward. As you breathe out, relax your diaphragm, allowing your belly to move back in. Practise this for 20 breaths. Your right hand should not move at all during this process.

05 Remove your hands and spend a minute observing how your breath continues to move your abdomen.

06 Conclude the practice whenever you are ready. Observe how you are feeling and notice how this is different to how you felt before.

"The way you breathe for the rest of your life will be more healthy, calming, and refreshing."

HAND SIGNALS

Using the mudras

You've learnt the art of sitting, but what do you do with your hands? Some meditators adopt hand postures called *mudras*, a Sanskrit word meaning "gesture", "attitude", or "seal".

There are hundreds of different *mudras*, each with a specific purpose, and they are used in many contemplative traditions within Buddhism and Yoga. Yogis believe that they have a subtle effect on the mind, although it is said that only advanced practitioners with sensitive awareness can notice it.

The five most common *mudras* used for meditation are shown here. As with everything else, it's best to experiment and see how each one feels for you. If you prefer, you can simply allow your hands to rest on your lap or knees.

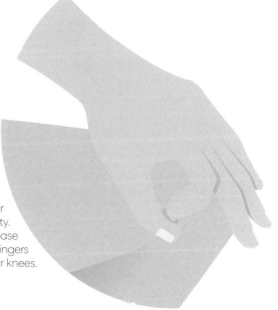

GESTURE OF CONSCIOUSNESS *(Chin mudra)*
The same position as *Jnana mudra* (below), but with your palms facing up. Both represent the union of the universal and individual consciousness. *Chin mudra* creates openness and receptivity, though it is harder to hold once your body relaxes.

" *Mudras are said to aid concentration and build up energy.*"

GESTURE OF KNOWLEDGE *(Jnana mudra)*
This *mudra* helps you connect to deeper wisdom and knowledge, and find clarity. Touch the tips of your index fingers to the base or tips of your thumbs. Stretch your other fingers out. Place your hands palms-down on your knees.

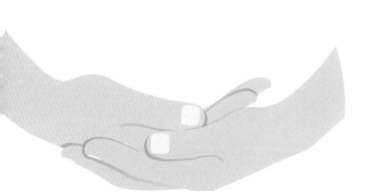

GESTURE OF MEDITATION (*Dhyana mudra*)
Also called *Yoga mudra* and *Samadhi mudra*, this is the preferred hand position for Buddhist meditation. It is thought to improve your ability to heal and concentrate. Place your left hand on your lap, palm up, and place your right hand on top. Extend your fingers and touch your thumbs together.

FIERCE GESTURE (*Bhairava mudra*)
This hand position stimulates inner strength, good health, and harmony in your energy flow. It is similar to *Dhyana mudra* (above right), but with the thumbs resting down.

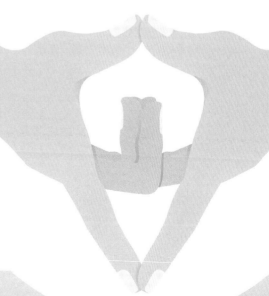

GESTURE OF THE WOMB (*Yoni mudra*)
Practised to calm and balance the nervous system and to bring stability and serenity, *Yoni mudra* helps move your awareness inside. Interlace your middle, ring, and little fingers so their pads touch. Touch your thumbs together and point your index fingers down.

THE ART OF CONCENTRATION

Balancing effort and relaxation

We all use some level of concentration in our daily lives, but rarely do we practise the intensity of focus needed in meditation. A deep state of concentration requires the balance of two things: effort and relaxation.

With too much effort in meditation you become tense and restless, but with too much relaxation you become drowsy and lazy. Deep concentration falls somewhere between the two: the right type of effort and the right type of relaxation, in the right balance.

To generate the right type of relaxation, let go of tensions in your body and mind, consciously "open up" and "sink in", but remain alert moment by moment. For the right type of effort, you need to create an internal feeling of intensity, but one that also has a sense of continuity, stability, and gentleness. It can help to generate a feeling of importance and interest towards your meditation, and to keep your interest alive. Imagining a metaphor of intensity will help you to channel this feeling (see opposite).

"*Getting the right balance will help you enter a state of flow.*"

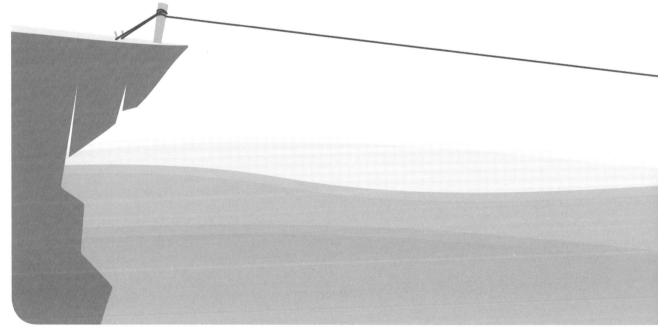

METAPHORS OF INTENSITY

These visual ideas aim to give the mind a sense of what intense unwavering presence feels like, which you can then apply to your meditation. When you do, you will enter the state of flow. This means you temporarily forget about yourself, your posture, and your environment, and become one with the object of your focus.

Meditate like…

● **A person on a tightrope** carefully placing foot after foot in perfect balance.

● **An artist carving a figure** on a matchstick, keeping their mind, eyes, and hand perfectly still.

● **A candle flame burning** steadily in a still room.

● **A cat patiently and quietly waiting** outside a hole, poised to pounce on a mouse.

● **A parent joyously hugging a child** they haven't seen for years.

● **Your mind is made of iron filings** and the object of your meditation is a powerful magnet.

● **Every drop of your being** has nowhere to go but with the meditation object.

● **Your mind is an arrow** flying towards a target.

● **You are placing a fence** around your mind so it can focus on only one thing, such as your breath.

● **Your hair is on fire** and the object of your meditation is water.

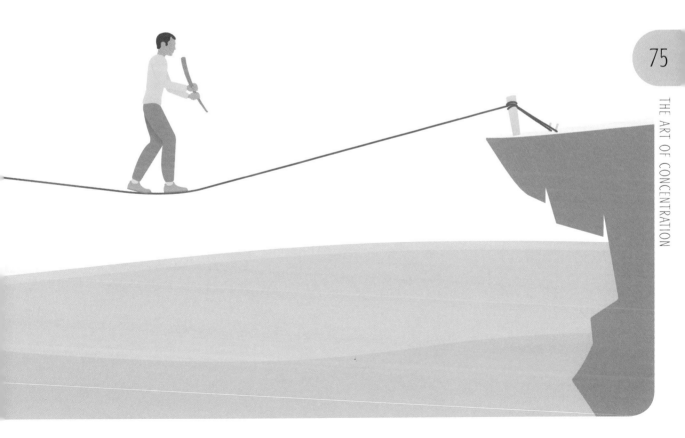

ANXIETY AND MEDITATION

When relaxing makes you restless

Meditation can help manage anxiety, but what if relaxation itself is a source of anxiety? If you experience relaxation-induced anxiety, the steps shown here will help you start to tackle it, but it's a good idea to consult a professional to have full support.

It helps to begin by understanding exactly what about relaxation is triggering anxiety for you. It is often a troublesome thought (see opposite), or a repressed emotion that, in the stillness and openness of meditation, starts to surface to the conscious mind. Whatever it is, recognize it fully and clearly.

ADJUSTING YOUR ATTITUDE

When you have clarity about what is causing your anxiety, you can start to consciously change your attitude towards relaxation. Next time you meditate, check in with your body, breath, and mind. Identify where in your body the anxiety is living: is it a sense of nervousness in your legs? A vibration around your chest? A pressure inside your head? Identify the exact sensations and tensions associated with the anxiety. Consciously relax these sensations with every exhalation.

Carefully observe the pattern of your breathing, and see how it is associated with your feelings of anxiety. Make sure your breath is abdominal, long, and slow (see pp.70–71).

If you're still struggling with an anxious thought, you can try practising affirmations that counter them (see opposite). If that doesn't help, simply know that relaxation and stillness might be uncomfortable at first. Accept the feeling of discomfort, any nervousness that arises, and the anxious thought patterns. Observe them as an uninvolved witness. Try to:

● **Let these feelings** and thoughts exist – allow them to come and go. Whatever they are, try not to be bothered by them. Just watch them.

● **Avoid creating** stories around these thoughts and feelings. There is no need to panic. Just keep watching, breathing, and letting go. The thoughts can't hurt you.

TRY SOMETHING DIFFERENT

Finally, if you're still facing anxiety, try shortening your sessions. It may help to experiment with more dynamic techniques such as Kinhin (see pp.90–91), Yoga Asanas (see pp.94–95), Tai Chi (see pp.96–97), or Humming Bee Pranayama (see pp.88–89).

"If relaxing makes you restless, it may help to know you are not alone."

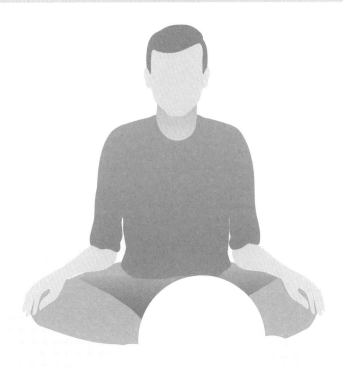

REFRAME YOUR THINKING

Relaxation anxiety often comes from an annoying thought, such as those shown below.
If, after calming your body and breath, you are still bothered by an anxious thought,
try practising affirmations that are the opposite of that thought.

ANXIOUS THOUGHTS

"I'm wasting my time."

"My body is too quiet and my breath
is too deep... This is scary!"

"What are these weird sensations
I'm having? Is this normal? Am I
doing it right?"

AFFIRMATIONS

 "Meditation is a great use of my time!"

 "I relax and let go inside this stillness. It is
peaceful, pleasant, nourishing, and reassuring."

 "Whatever is happening, it's okay.
I am safe. I am the witness of
all these sensations."

THE MANY TYPES OF MEDITATION

YOUR OWN PATH

Finding a practice that works for you

In this chapter, you'll be introduced to a number of different meditation techniques. It may seem hard to know which to try first, but taking some time to reflect and explore is a great first step.

The meditations shown in this chapter are the most popular techniques from the main traditions, and they can all be practised in a secular way. They are grouped by which sensory channel they use most, starting with those that use all channels simultaneously, followed by body and sensation, breath, sight, sound, mind, and heart. These different approaches have developed over time to suit our different needs, personalities, and goals, all of which can change throughout our lives. While many techniques share several benefits – such as reducing stress and worry (see pp.24–27) – each has its own unique characteristics, "feel", and results, so it is important to choose one that works for you.

GROUP PRACTICE

You can practise all of the meditations in this chapter on your own at home. However, some people find it beneficial to meditate with a teacher or in a group. For example, it is said that Transcendental Meditation, or TM, can only be learned from a teacher authorized by the TM organization. For this reason, it is not covered in this chapter. Another unique and important technique not shown here is Kirtan chanting, as it is best practised as part of a group (see pp.178–179).

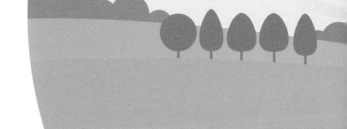

THE THREE KEY SKILLS

Meditation involves awareness, relaxation, and concentration. These skills are essentially present, in one form or another, in all techniques. However, each style of meditation tends to develop one skill more than the others, and this is something you may want to take into account when choosing your technique.

The Key Facts box for each technique in this chapter indicates which skill it develops the most. This can help you understand the difference between the practices, though it is worth bearing in mind that some techniques could fit into more than one category.

"Your meditation experience and the effects it has on you depend on the technique you choose."

CHOOSING A TECHNIQUE

There is only one way: self-experimentation. No technique is universally "the best" for everyone as we are all different. Following the steps below will help you work out which style best works for you, according to your temperament, needs, and goals.

Start by working out what you most want from meditation: What are the benefits you seek most? Stress relief? Getting in touch with your inner self? Improving memory and concentration? Are you more of a body, mind, or heart person? What experiences or feelings do you most value in a meditation practice? Peace? Equanimity? Love and connection? Stillness? Clarity and insight? Groundedness? Which skill do you want to develop the most? Awareness, relaxation, or concentration (see opposite)?

Read through the techniques in this chapter and try any that you feel some attraction towards for three to four days each. Keep a journal of the results.

Narrow down to two to four techniques you want to explore further. Practise each technique for another two weeks to one month.

Learn more about these techniques and, if you can, talk to other people who practise or teach them.

Finally, choose one core technique for your daily practice. You can still practise other techniques from time to time, but keeping largely with one technique will help you go deeper with it.

MINDFULNESS MEDITATION

Present moment awareness

Mindfulness Meditation practises the skill of non-judgmental awareness, meaning that you hold things in view without creating unnecessary reactions towards them. This is a popular seated meditation, which includes different elements of mindfulness.

WHY CHOOSE THIS PRACTICE?

Mindfulness is one of the most popular meditation practices in the West and it is very secular by nature. It's a simple way to become more grounded in the present moment and develop a non-judgmental awareness about how your body and mind work.

Imagine it is raining, for example, and you have forgotten your umbrella. You feel your body tense up and you become annoyed or upset. With mindfulness, you simply notice the rain and become aware that your body is tensing up and your mind is spinning thoughts of complaint. You don't run blindly with any of these thoughts and you don't create layers of interpretations about them. This accepting, raw, non-judgmental awareness is mindfulness.

KEY FACTS

• **Essence** Moment-by-moment non-judgmental awareness of whatever arises in your body and mind, with an anchor of breathing

• **Sensory channel** Multi-channel, breath

• **Skill** Awareness

• **Tradition** Buddhism, secular

• **Similar practices** Mini-meditation 3, Vipassana, Inner Silence, Labelling, Zazen

01 Sit in a stable and comfortable meditation posture. You can keep your eyes open or close them. Take three deep breaths through your nose. Relax your body with every out-breath.

02 Bring your attention to your breathing and gently rest it there. Even when noticing other things – such as the sounds in your environment, sensations in your body, and any thoughts that arise – always keep part of your attention with the breath.

08 Whenever you are ready, gently move your body and conclude the practice.

07 Finally, notice your mind. Your mind will keep producing thoughts. Be aware of the thoughts coming and going, but don't latch onto any of them. Continue noticing everything, without holding onto anything. Keep your breathing as the anchor throughout your practice.

" Whenever you realize that your mind has wandered, simply notice that, and gently bring the awareness back to the breath."

06 Then, notice any sensations in your body, for example, pain and pleasure, heat and coolness, or tension and relaxation.

05 First, notice your environment. When sounds come through your ears, you notice them as they are. You also notice if they create any reactions in you and you accept those as well.

03 You can observe the sensations of the air coming in and out of your nostrils, or how breathing moves your chest or belly. Or you can count your breaths with every exhalation, from 10 to 1, to help you stay present.

04 You can stay with the breath, or choose to take it further. To do this, you'll open your awareness up to your environment, body, and mind, always keeping the breath as an anchor. Whatever arises is seen with non-judgmental awareness.

ZAZEN

Just Sitting, here and now

Zazen can involve concentrating on the breath, contemplating a question, statement, or riddle (a *koan*), or Just Sitting (*shikantaza*), as shown here. Just Sitting has no object, and is a form of open present moment awareness.

WHY CHOOSE THIS PRACTICE?

Zazen emphasizes physical posture as a frame to keep the mind present, open, and aware. In the form of Just Sitting, shown here, Zazen helps you develop a panoramic awareness of your mind and life. A very simple and direct meditation, it is based on the idea that the ultimate reality already is as it is. Every being is already a realized Buddha, and the practice of Just Sitting is simply an actualization of your inherent Buddhahood. The steps shown here are just guidelines to help you find the right state of mind for the practice.

KEY FACTS

- **Essence** Panoramic awareness of the present moment. Simply sit and let go of thinking
- **Sensory channel** Multi-channel, breath
- **Skill** Awareness, concentration
- **Tradition** Buddhism, particularly Zen Buddhism
- **Similar practices** Mindfulness, Vipassana

84

01 Sit in an upright position, with your back and neck straight and unsupported, facing a wall. Position your hands in *Dhyana mudra* (see p.73). Your ears should be in line with your shoulders and your nose in line with your navel.

02 Place your tongue against the roof of your mouth and keep it closed. Your eyes should be half open, with your gaze resting on the floor or the wall in front of you.

03 Release all thoughts in an attitude of non-thinking and let everything be as it is. Relax in the now, and keep a panoramic awareness of everything that arises in your consciousness, without zooming in on anything. This is called dropping off body and mind.

05 Don't analyze or conceptualize. Just sit and be with what is. When thoughts arise, let them pass like clouds in the sky.

06 Remain alert: don't fall into sleep, and don't drift into thinking. Simply keep returning your attention to the pose and the panoramic and detached awareness of the here and now.

04 Let your awareness spread through your whole body, mind, and environment. Allow everything to be noticed, but don't cling to or reject anything.

07 Sit in Zazen without any goals, or thoughts of gaining anything from your practice. Let go of all expectation and desire, and remain open and present to reality as it is. Zazen is not meant to achieve anything, or to be a special experience. It is not a means to an end.

08 When you're ready, bend forward in gratitude for the practice with folded hands, and slowly move out of Zazen.

"Don't engage with your thoughts and don't suppress them. Simply notice them passively and non-judgmentally."

VIPASSANA

Insight into impermanence

Vipassana is a Pali word meaning "clear seeing" or "insight". It is one of the two original Buddhist meditations alongside Samatha. Concentration is the basis of Vipassana, not its goal – its goal is insight, awareness, and letting go.

WHY CHOOSE THIS PRACTICE?

Vipassana's main aim is not to calm and relax, but to develop insight into the nature of your mind, body, and sensations, and to awaken to the reality of things as they are. As the practice deepens, a true restructuring of the personality, sense of self, and view of the world takes place.

As with all meditations, there are variations in this practice. The one shown here is closest to the teachings of Vipassana Movement, which includes mindfulness of thoughts and feelings alongside breathing awareness. Its emphasis is on seeing the three marks of existence – impermanence, suffering, and non-self – in all things.

KEY FACTS

- **Essence** Seeking insight into the nature of the mind and all phenomena, understanding its impermanence, and letting go

- **Sensory channel** Multi-channel, breath

- **Skill** Awareness

- **Tradition** Buddhism

- **Similar practices** Mindfulness, Zazen, Inner Silence, Labelling

02 Bring your attention to the sensations of breathing, particularly the rise and fall of your abdomen and chest. Witness every movement of breath with full attention. After some time, move your attention to the sensation of the breath moving through your nostrils. If you realize that you have lost awareness of the breath, notice that fact, and gently bring it back.

01 Sit in a meditation posture and close your eyes. Take three deep breaths through your nose. Relax your body with every out-breath.

03 Scan your body for sensations, such as heat or cold, tension or relaxation, lightness or heaviness. Let your attention rest on each for some time. Observe how it is impermanent and in constant flux. See if it is perceived as pleasant, unpleasant, or neutral, but don't react to it – simply observe it as it is. Go deep inside each sensation and try to find its essence.

04 Move your attention to the world of the mind. Observe mental phenomena that arise, such as thoughts, feelings, memories, desires, and states of mind. Watch them arise and pass away. Refrain from engaging with them or rejecting them.

05 Notice how the thoughts are impermanent, fleeting, and in constant flux. The moment you try to grab hold of them, they are gone. Zoom into the thoughts and try to find their essence. In the same way, observe and investigate the general states of your mind – active or lethargic, distracted or composed, bright or dull.

"You are aware of your thoughts, but you are not thinking the thoughts."

06 When you are ready, slowly start moving your fingers, open your eyes, and conclude the practice.

HUMMING BEE PRANAYAMA

The sound of silence

Pranayama is a breathing exercise in the Yogic tradition which can serve as a preparation for meditation, as well as a practice in its own right. The Humming Bee Pranayama (also called *bhramari*) is a technique that calms the mind and turns your awareness inside.

WHY CHOOSE THIS PRACTICE?

There are many health and wellbeing benefits to practising pranayama, including reducing stress and anxiety, and relieving anger or frustration.

In Humming Bee Pranayama, the practice becomes meditative when, after finishing the breathing, you listen for subtle sounds in your body and consciousness. The vibration of the "hum" sound pacifies the brain and nervous system, improves concentration, and gives a cooling feeling. Don't practise this pranayama if you have tinnitus or an ear infection.

02 Take three deep breaths through your nose. With every out-breath your body gets more relaxed and still. Close your mouth, but keep your teeth apart.

01 Sit still in a comfortable meditation posture. Close your eyes.

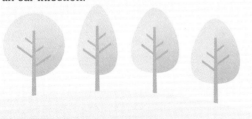

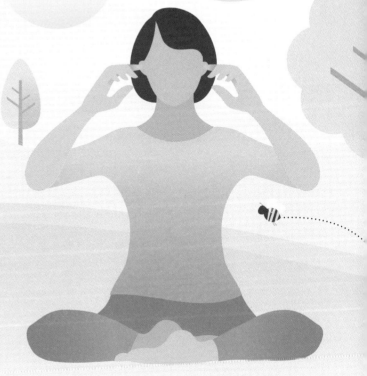

KEY FACTS

- **Essence** A rhythmic breathing exercise to calm the body and mind

- **Sensory channel** Breath

- **Skill** Relaxation, awareness

- **Tradition** Yoga, specifically part of Nada Yoga, or yoga of sound

- **Similar practices** Alternate nostril breathing

04 Inhale slowly through your nose, then exhale slowly, making a continuous, smooth humming sound, like a drawn out "hum". Feel the vibrations in your head and chest. Practise 7 rounds, then do another 3 while making the "hum" in your mind, with no audible sound.

05 Relax your arms on your lap. Keep your eyes closed and stay in the posture. Let go of repeating the sound in your mind. Now, try to hear internal sounds in your body or mind. Imagine your whole being is an ear and turn it inside.

03 Close both your ears with your thumbs or index fingers. Keep your elbows raised (see below).

06 You may hear a humming sound, a white noise, your heartbeat, or nothing at all. It doesn't matter which. If you do hear any subtle sounds, then focus your mind on them. If not, just keep listening, with no expectation and infinite patience.

07 Pay attention to your body. Feel the contact of your body with the floor, stool, or chair. Bring your attention to the breath and notice it as it is. When you are ready, slowly move your body, open your eyes, and come out of the meditation.

hmmmmmmmmmm

"It doesn't matter if you don't hear anything – the key is to develop receptivity."

HUMMING BEE PRANAYAMA

KINHIN

Walking Zen

Kinhin, also known as "Walking Zen", is a form of dynamic meditation in which you keep your concentration on the breath, in synchronization with each step. Only a small part of your awareness is with the environment.

WHY CHOOSE THIS PRACTICE?

As a more active meditation technique, Kinhin is particularly good for people who find it hard to sit still. It is also popular at meditation retreats, as it allows the legs to rest in between seated meditation sessions.

In some Zen schools the pace is very slow (half a step with every full breath), while in others it is much quicker (several steps with each breath). The slower method is shown here, but you can experiment with speeds and rhythms to see how they affect your mind.

KEY FACTS

- **Essence** Walking meditation with a focus on deep breathing
- **Sensory channel** Breath, body and sensation
- **Skill** Concentration
- **Tradition** Buddhism, particularly Zen
- **Similar practices** Zazen, Mindfulness, Tai Chi

04 Imagine that the top of your head is being pulled gently towards the sky by a thread. This will help to keep your neck straight.

03 Adopt the *Shashu* position for your hands (see opposite).

02 Relax your body, while keeping it upright. You should feel stable but relaxed.

01 Stand up straight, with your feet hip-width apart, and weight evenly distributed between both legs.

"Keep the body aligned, stable, and upright throughout the whole practice."

05 Gaze about five or six feet in front of you, without focusing on anything in particular. Relax the muscles on your face, shoulders, and hips.

06 With each out-breath, take half a step forward, starting with the right foot (see below). Pay full attention to your breath and steps.

07 As in seated meditation, let thoughts come and go, but keep bringing your attention back to the breath. When you are ready, slowly bow in respect to the practice, raise your eyes, and walk away.

Form a fist with your left hand by wrapping your fingers around your thumb.

Move your elbows away from your body, so that they form a line and are parallel to the floor.

Wrap your right hand around your left hand so that the thumb of the right hand rests near the bottom of the thumb of the left hand.

Place both hands in line with your navel, or with the centre of the chest.

Posture principles
Follow the guidelines above to adopt the *Shashu* hand position, or *mudra*. Make sure that you feel stable, straight, relaxed, and comfortable (see p.67).

Take half a step forward each time, so your heel will replace the tips of your toes.

YOGA NIDRA

Body scans and deep relaxation

Based on a Tantric practice, this variation of Yoga Nidra uses a body scan and visualization to achieve a state of deep relaxation. It can help to follow a guided meditation audio.

WHY CHOOSE THIS PRACTICE?

Yoga Nidra aims to release all tensions (whether muscular, emotional, or mental), develop awareness of unconscious states of mind, and prepare the mind for the states of deep meditation. It also seeks to bring about personal transformation by establishing a resolution (*sankalpa*) deep in your subconscious. Before you start, choose your resolution – this is a short, clear, and affirmative sentence that expresses a commitment for your life. It is best to always use the same one until it gets fulfilled in you.

KEY FACTS

• **Essence** A lying-down meditation that involves a body scan, setting a resolution, and visualizations

• **Sensory channel** Body and sensation

• **Skill** Relaxation, awareness

• **Tradition** Yoga

• **Similar practices** Mindfulness, Mini-meditation 1

02 Pay attention to the sounds in your environment for a few moments. Stay with each sound for a few seconds, without judging it, then move on to the next.

01 Lie down with your back and neck aligned, feet hip-width apart, arms stretched out, and palms facing up. You can place a thin cushion under your neck and a blanket over your body. Then, close your eyes and surrender your body to the floor. Have the intention of not falling asleep and of keeping your body still throughout.

"Your resolution will go deep into your subconscious mind, so choose it carefully."

03 Become aware of the contact of your body with the floor: the heels, backs of the legs, buttocks, upper back, arms, and head.

04 Repeat your resolution in your mind three times. Say it slowly, with full conviction and intention. Let it sink deep inside.

05 Move your awareness through each part of your body one by one, saying its name in your mind and "feeling into it" for 2–3 seconds. For example, start with the toes of your right foot, then move through the sole, top of the foot, heel, ankle, lower leg, knee, upper leg, and buttock. Then repeat for the left foot and leg.

06 Continue this process, moving up through your abdomen, chest, back, each hand and arm, then neck, head, and face. Next, become aware of larger parts of your body, such as both legs and feet, whole torso, arms and hands. Finally, move your awareness to your whole body.

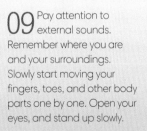

07 Bring your awareness back to the breath. Observe it as it is, then count your breaths from 20 to 1. After this, say your resolution three times, with intention and conviction.

08 When you're ready, become aware of the contact of your body with the floor again. Notice how your breath moves your body. Deepen your breath a little and notice how this brings movement to your body.

09 Pay attention to external sounds. Remember where you are and your surroundings. Slowly start moving your fingers, toes, and other body parts one by one. Open your eyes, and stand up slowly.

YOGA ASANAS

Stillness from pose to pose

Many people think that Yoga is simply about stretching and elaborate poses, or asanas, but asanas can be a dynamic form of meditation in their own right. Asanas are good for short meditations, or in preparation for seated practices.

WHY CHOOSE THIS PRACTICE?

Yoga Asanas work well as a meditation for people who are very connected to the body, have a more dynamic nature, and find it hard to sit still. Start with more accessible asanas, such as those shown here, as this helps you relax and focus. Each of these poses also practises a key element of meditation – concentration, awareness, and relaxation.

To practise Yoga Asanas as meditation, bring your attention fully to your body and breath, and move in and out of each pose slowly and mindfully. In your final pose, relax deeply and stay still, without stiffness or tension, for a few minutes if you are practising one or two poses, or at least 60 seconds if you are practising more. If you have health concerns, consult a doctor first.

KEY FACTS

- **Essence** Learning to deeply relax and find stillness in different postures
- **Sensory channel** Body and sensation, breath
- **Skill** Relaxation, awareness
- **Tradition** Yoga
- **Similar practices** Tai Chi, Kinhin

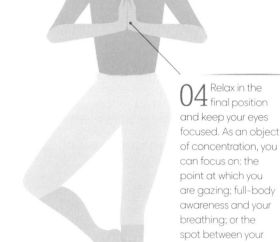

01 Stand up tall, and focus your gaze on a point ahead of you. This facilitates balance and concentration.

03 Bring both of your hands together in front of your chest. If this is too easy, raise them above your head.

04 Relax in the final position and keep your eyes focused. As an object of concentration, you can focus on: the point at which you are gazing; full-body awareness and your breathing; or the spot between your eyebrows (the Third Eye chakra).

02 Bend one leg and place the sole of your foot on your lower leg, below the knee. To make it harder, place it on the inside of your thigh.

TREE POSE (*Vrikshasana*)
Balancing in this asana helps you concentrate, so if you find it too easy, you can adjust the pose to make it harder (see above). To balance, you also need relaxation, full-body awareness, and mental calmness, all of which help your meditation.

01 Lie down straight on your front.

02 Raise the upper part of your body, place your elbows on the floor, and relax your head on your hands.

03 Your big toes should touch each other, but let your feet fall to the sides.

04 Gaze into the void in front of you. Let your eyes be still and fully relaxed. There is nowhere to focus, so the eyes and mind are resting in emptiness. Dwell on that awareness.

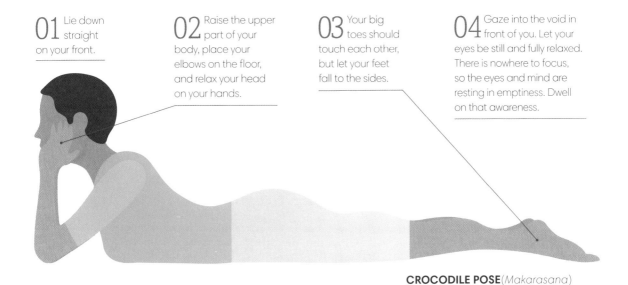

CROCODILE POSE (*Makarasana*)
To develop your awareness in this pose, focus on "just being" while keeping your awareness open and detached. For relaxation, focus on the body and feeling your muscles stretch and release.

01 Kneel on the floor, sitting on your heels, with your legs and knees touching.

02 Lower your torso, until your forehead is touching the floor.

03 Place your arms beside your legs, palms upwards, with your hands by your feet.

04 Close your eyes. Relax your shoulders, back, legs, and arms.

05 Let go of all tensions. With every out-breath, relax even more.

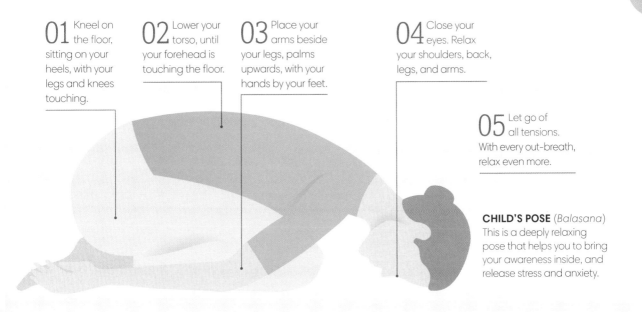

CHILD'S POSE (*Balasana*)
This is a deeply relaxing pose that helps you to bring your awareness inside, and release stress and anxiety.

TAI CHI

Standing Like a Tree

Tai Chi (*taijiquan*) is a Chinese martial art of Taoist origin. Originally practised as self-defence, Tai Chi is now used to cultivate good health and body-mind harmony. Standing Like a Tree (*zhan zhuang*) works well for meditation.

WHY CHOOSE THIS PRACTICE?

The slow, focused movements of Tai Chi are thought to relieve stress, develop mental clarity, and help you experience a sense of calmness and fluidity in movement. Tai Chi also grounds you in your body, and improves your flexibility and balance.

Standing Like a Tree was first created to promote health, develop internal power, and help the flow of energy (*qi*) in the body. There is a lot to pay attention to, which helps you focus on the present. You can hold this pose for 1–10 minutes. By keeping still for extended periods of time while focusing on the breath, you feel a sense of vitality building up in your body and mind. Your body can feel so perfectly balanced, stable, and whole that you don't want to move a single muscle. In that there is peace, clarity, and great inner strength.

03 Keep your spine and neck straight. Imagine that the top of your head is slightly being pulled towards the ceiling by an invisible string.

02 Crouch slightly, bending your knees, so they reach no further than the line of your toes. Roll your pelvis back slightly, so your lower back is softly rounded.

01 Stand up straight with your feet about hip-width apart, parallel, and pointing forward. Stretch your toes and feel as though you are grasping the ground with them.

KEY FACTS

- **Essence** Holding a still and balanced posture to still and balance the mind

- **Sensory channel** Body and sensation, breath

- **Skill** Relaxation

- **Tradition** Taoism

- **Similar practices** Yoga Asanas, Kinhin

"*Body and mind are both soft and stable at the same time, both relaxed and alert.*"

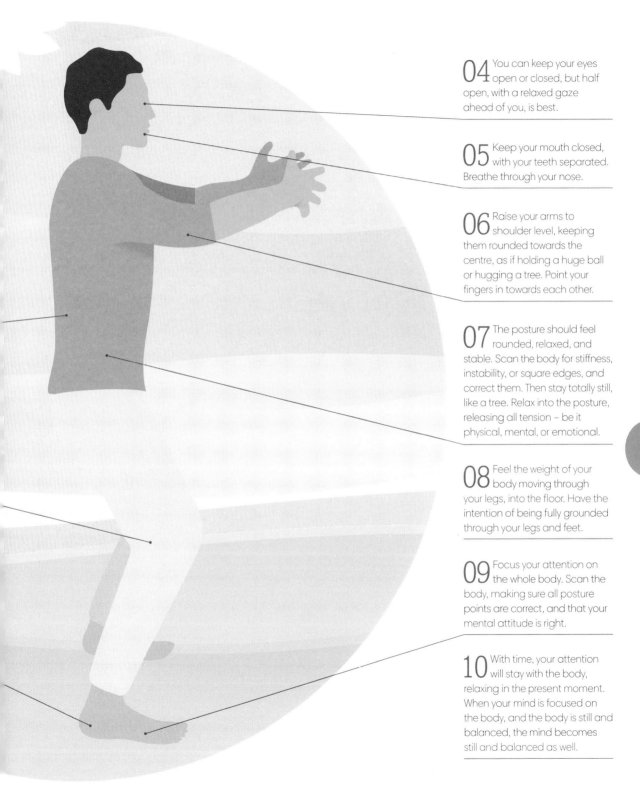

04 You can keep your eyes open or closed, but half open, with a relaxed gaze ahead of you, is best.

05 Keep your mouth closed, with your teeth separated. Breathe through your nose.

06 Raise your arms to shoulder level, keeping them rounded towards the centre, as if holding a huge ball or hugging a tree. Point your fingers in towards each other.

07 The posture should feel rounded, relaxed, and stable. Scan the body for stiffness, instability, or square edges, and correct them. Then stay totally still, like a tree. Relax into the posture, releasing all tension – be it physical, mental, or emotional.

08 Feel the weight of your body moving through your legs, into the floor. Have the intention of being fully grounded through your legs and feet.

09 Focus your attention on the whole body. Scan the body, making sure all posture points are correct, and that your mental attitude is right.

10 With time, your attention will stay with the body, relaxing in the present moment. When your mind is focused on the body, and the body is still and balanced, the mind becomes still and balanced as well.

NEIGUAN

An inner exploration of the body

Developed around the 7th or 8th century, Neiguan is one of the five main Taoist meditation practices. It is an elaborate exercise involving the visualization and "feeling" of your body from the inside. The technique shown here is a simplified adaptation.

WHY CHOOSE THIS PRACTICE?

In Neiguan, you feel and visualize the five main organs of traditional Chinese medicine, each of which is connected to a colour, emotion, and one of the five elements in Chinese philosophy. As a result, Neiguan helps you connect to your body in a deeper way. If no specific images come to mind, just have the intention of wanting to see. You can practise this technique by yourself, but if you want to take it further, it is best to join a Taoist group.

KEY FACTS

- **Essence** Visualizing and feeling your body from the inside
- **Sensory channel** Body and sensation, sight
- **Skill** Awareness
- **Tradition** Taoism
- **Similar practices** Visualization, Yoga Nidra, Kundalini

02 Spend a minute centring your attention in your body. Allow your mind to settle too. Then, start feeling your body from the inside. Take a couple of minutes to develop the sensitivity, then open the "eye of your mind" so you can both feel and see your body from the inside.

01 Sit still in a comfortable posture. Close your eyes and take three deep breaths through your nose. Let your body become relaxed and still with every out-breath.

"Don't think too much about each step. Approach it with an open mind."

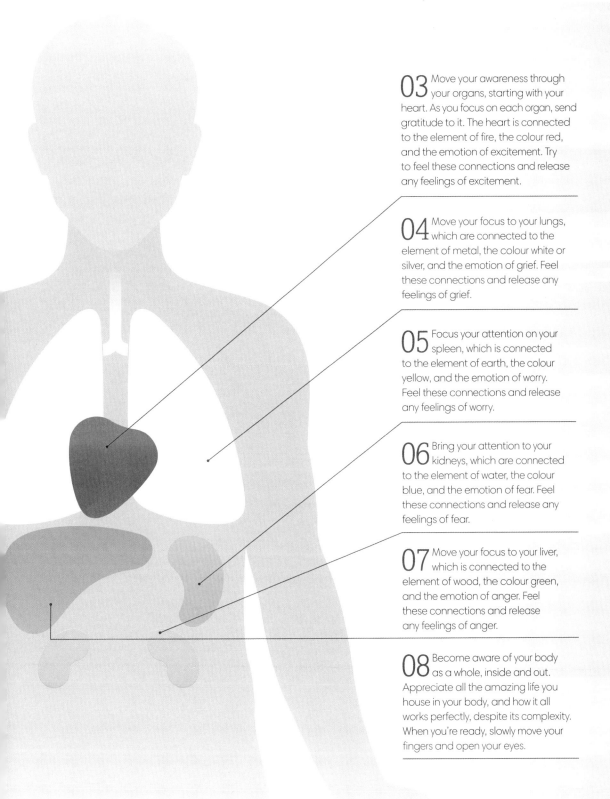

03 Move your awareness through your organs, starting with your heart. As you focus on each organ, send gratitude to it. The heart is connected to the element of fire, the colour red, and the emotion of excitement. Try to feel these connections and release any feelings of excitement.

04 Move your focus to your lungs, which are connected to the element of metal, the colour white or silver, and the emotion of grief. Feel these connections and release any feelings of grief.

05 Focus your attention on your spleen, which is connected to the element of earth, the colour yellow, and the emotion of worry. Feel these connections and release any feelings of worry.

06 Bring your attention to your kidneys, which are connected to the element of water, the colour blue, and the emotion of fear. Feel these connections and release any feelings of fear.

07 Move your focus to your liver, which is connected to the element of wood, the colour green, and the emotion of anger. Feel these connections and release any feelings of anger.

08 Become aware of your body as a whole, inside and out. Appreciate all the amazing life you house in your body, and how it all works perfectly, despite its complexity. When you're ready, slowly move your fingers and open your eyes.

KUNDALINI

Serpent power and the chakras

Kundalini refers to the psycho-spiritual energy lying at the bottom of the spine, where the root chakra (*muladhara*) lies. Here, you move your consciousness through the chakras, following a specific mantra and visualization for each.

WHY CHOOSE THIS PRACTICE?

Kundalini means "coiled" and it is symbolically represented by a coiled snake. The goal of this practice is to purify the body and mind, activate and purify the chakras (energy centres), awaken the Kundalini energy, and make it rise through the chakras all the way to the crown of the head. The meditation shown here is one of several Kundalini practices and is a simplified version. Traditionally, it is a very complex art, so it is best to seek expert guidance before practising this meditation. Otherwise, keep your sessions short, and stop the practice if you feel any negative effects.

KEY FACTS

- **Essence** Moving the mind through the different chakras in the body, including the use of visualizations and mantras

- **Sensory channel** Body and sensation, sight, sound

- **Skill** Concentration

- **Tradition** Yoga, specifically Tantra Yoga and Kriya Yoga

- **Similar practices** Third Eye Meditation, Mantra, Visualization

01 Sit still in a comfortable meditation posture. Close your eyes and take three deep breaths through your nose. Let your body become relaxed and still with every out-breath. Focus on your whole body for a few minutes, until the mind settles.

04 Focus on the **SOLAR PLEXUS** chakra. Visualize a blazing yellow sun shining there. Repeat the mantra "*ram*".

03 Focus on the **SACRAL** chakra. Visualize a crescent moon there. Repeat the mantra "*vam*".

02 Focus on the **ROOT** chakra. Visualize a red inverted triangle there. Repeat the mantra "*lam*".

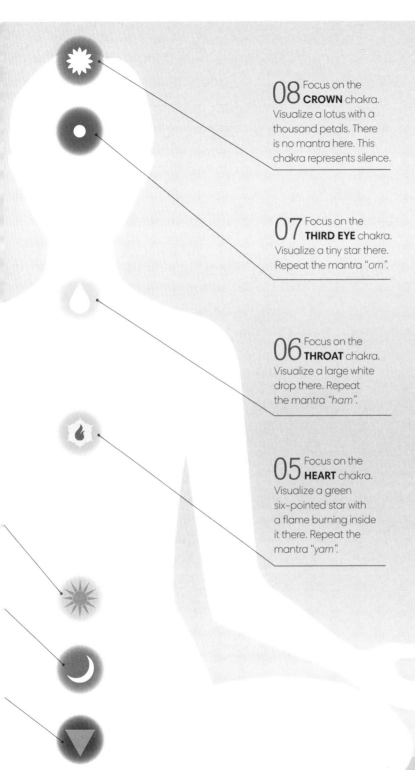

08 Focus on the **CROWN** chakra. Visualize a lotus with a thousand petals. There is no mantra here. This chakra represents silence.

09 Slowly bring your attention back down to the root chakra, passing through the seven chakras one by one, while repeating their mantra three times.

07 Focus on the **THIRD EYE** chakra. Visualize a tiny star there. Repeat the mantra "*om*".

10 Become aware of your whole body and the movement of your breath for a few moments. Then, slowly move your fingers, open your eyes, and conclude the practice.

06 Focus on the **THROAT** chakra. Visualize a large white drop there. Repeat the mantra "*ham*".

05 Focus on the **HEART** chakra. Visualize a green six-pointed star with a flame burning inside it there. Repeat the mantra "*yam*".

TRATAKA

The power of gazing

Gazing steadily, without moving the pupils, is a powerful way to still the mind and develop strong concentration. As with mantra and breathing, gazing meditation is found in many contemplative traditions. The technique shown here is from the Yogic tradition and uses a candle as its object.

03 When you are relaxed, gently open your eyes and let them rest at the top of the wick. Relax your eye muscles fully and keep them steady.

01 In a dark room, place a candle in front of you at eye level, about two feet away. Ensure it is in a stable place, away from draughts. Sit still in a comfortable posture and close your eyes.

02 Take three deep breaths through your nose. Your body becomes more relaxed and still with every out-breath.

102

"Don't concentrate on not blinking. Instead, have the subtle intention of allowing the eyes to be relaxed and still."

WHY CHOOSE THIS PRACTICE?

Trataka develops concentration, focus, and visualization, and is a good foundation for other practices. It is easier to focus on luminous objects, like a candle flame or the moon, but you can select almost any object, such as a dot on the wall, an image, or a leaf. If you practise with a luminous object every day, take a break from the practice after two months to rest the eyes for 1–2 months. In the meantime, you can practise Trataka on a non-luminous object. You should also avoid using a candle if you have cataracts, glaucoma, myopia, astigmatism, or epilepsy.

KEY FACTS

- **Essence** Gazing steadily at an object, usually a candle flame
- **Sensory channel** Sight
- **Skill** Concentration
- **Tradition** Yoga
- **Similar practices** Mini-meditation 2, Third Eye Meditation

04 Let your whole awareness focus on the flame. Mind and eyes are one. Feel that the flame is all there is in the universe.

05 Close your eyes after about 3 minutes, or if they feel strained. With your eyes closed, keep staring in the same direction. You might see the after image of the candle. If you do, focus on it.

06 If the after image moves around, don't follow it. Just keep staring at the centre, with the intention of seeing it there. Even if it disappears, keep staring at where it was. It may come back.

07 Don't worry if you don't see anything, or if the after image quickly disappears. Just keep watching the black screen of your mind, and notice whatever appears.

08 When your eyes feel rested and you no longer see an after image, you can open your eyes and complete another round of outward and inward gazing.

09 To finish, rub your hands together and cup them over your closed eyes. Look down, then gently open your eyes. Let them rest gazing at the void for a few moments, then conclude the practice.

VISUALIZATION

Seeing with closed eyes

The ability to project and see forms clearly on the inside "screen" of your mind can be very challenging, but it is a powerful way to develop concentration. It is used as a meditation technique in many contemplative traditions.

WHY CHOOSE THIS PRACTICE?

Visualization practices strongly develop concentration and improve your memory and creativity. It can take a long time to feel that you've really made progress, but when mastered, the images you create in your mind will feel as real and sharp as the ones you see with your eyes.

This practice can be done anywhere, in any position, but you may find it easier to concentrate if you sit in a meditation posture and take a minute or two to relax your body and calm your breath first.

KEY FACTS

- **Essence** Creating and holding on to mental images
- **Sensory channel** Sight
- **Skill** Concentration
- **Tradition** Many, including Tibetan Buddhism, Yoga, and Taoism
- **Similar practices** Third Eye Meditation, Kundalini, Expand Your Consciousness

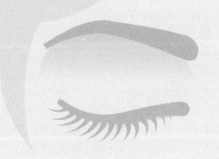
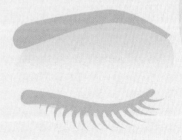

> *"The more your body and mind are relaxed and still, the easier it is to create steady images."*

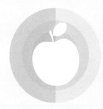

SCENERY

Here, you gradually add more images to a visualization. It helps to choose a scene without too many objects.

01 Open your eyes and observe an object in your field of vision for 1 minute.

02 Close your eyes and try to visualize that object, in the same size and position, on the screen of your mind. Try to hold it there for 1 minute.

03 Repeat this process two more times. Each time, add more detail, colour, and sharpness.

04 Without losing that first visualization, start to bring more objects into your mental field. Try introducing the object next to the first one, or the background landscape.

05 Gradually compose a mental image of everything you see when your eyes are open.

06 To finish, bring your attention back to your whole body. Observe your breathing for a few moments, then slowly move out of the posture and open your eyes.

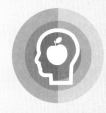

IMAGE RECALL

In this meditation, you replay a past event in your mind, adding as much detail as possible.

01 Close your eyes and think of something that happened to you today.

02 Try to visualize that event on the screen of your mind. Think of it as though you are watching it as a film, scene by scene.

03 See the people that were there, visualize their clothes and their facial expressions.

04 See the objects around you and what the lighting was like. See yourself as part of it, the posture of your body, and your clothes.

05 Spend some time composing that event in your mind and holding it as a single scene. Don't worry if you are doing this right or not.

06 To finish, bring your attention back to your whole body. Observe your breathing for a few moments, then slowly move out of the posture and open your eyes.

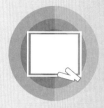

MENTAL BLACKBOARD

Visualize a blackboard and write on it in your mind. Remember to keep your mind still and relaxed.

01 Close your eyes and imagine a blackboard. Write words or numbers on the blackboard – they can be anything you like. Continue for about 5 minutes.

02 Start writing full sentences. You could use a quote you like, one of your thoughts, or an event from your day written as a narrative.

03 To finish, bring your attention back to your whole body. Observe your breathing for a few moments, then slowly move out of the posture and open your eyes.

MANDALA MEDITATION

Symbols for the subconscious mind

A mandala, such as the one shown right, is a geometrical symbol used in Yogic and Buddhist meditation to bypass the conscious mind and evoke experiences, feelings, and insight from your subconscious.

WHY CHOOSE THIS PRACTICE?

By accessing the subconscious mind, Mandala Meditation is believed to integrate deeper layers of your personality into your conscious life, and liberate you from repressed memories.

When choosing your mandala, select one that has the strongest appeal for you. If you find it hard to visualize mandalas with your eyes closed, drawing or colouring them – either freely, or following a guide – is a useful preparatory or contemplative exercise.

106

03 When you feel calm and centred, open your eyes and look at your mandala. Observe all the lines and objects in it. Explore all its corners. Appreciate its colours, shapes, and patterns.

02 Close your eyes for a few moments and take a few deep breaths, relaxing your body with each out-breath.

01 Sit comfortably in a meditation posture, facing your mandala. You can either hold it on a piece of paper or hang it on a wall.

KEY FACTS

- **Essence** Contemplating sacred symbols as a way to access the subconscious mind
- **Sensory channel** Sight, mind
- **Skill** Awareness
- **Tradition** Yoga, Buddhism
- **Similar practices** Yoga Nidra, Kundalini, Trataka

"Don't try to understand or interpret the mandala: simply explore it with curiosity and amazement."

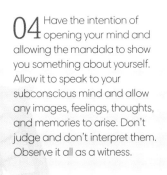

04 Have the intention of opening your mind and allowing the mandala to show you something about yourself. Allow it to speak to your subconscious mind and allow any images, feelings, thoughts, and memories to arise. Don't judge and don't interpret them. Observe it all as a witness.

05 An optional continuation of the meditation is to rest your eyes at the centre of the mandala and gaze there continuously. This makes the practice more intense, and more concentrative in nature. Whenever your eyes get tired from gazing, close them and rest them for a while, before starting another round of gazing.

06 When you are ready, close your eyes and bring your awareness back to your body. Feel your body as a whole. Observe your breathing pattern. Then, open your eyes and conclude the practice.

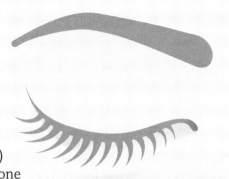

THIRD EYE MEDITATIONS

A door to superconsciousness

Of the seven main chakras (energy centres) in the body, the Third Eye (*ajna chakra*) is one of the most commonly used for meditation. The techniques shown here cover different ways of focusing your attention on this centre.

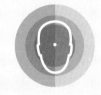

WHY CHOOSE THIS PRACTICE?

Meditating on the Third Eye is traditionally associated with discernment, wisdom, control of the mind, willpower, awakening of intuition, altered states of consciousness, transcending the ego, and purity. Whether you believe in its existence, or think it is symbolic, many people find that these meditations have a powerful effect on the mind.

Don't raise the eyes too much and don't strain, as this can cause headaches. If any of these techniques trigger confusing or unpleasant experiences, consult a meditation teacher.

KEY FACTS

- **Essence** Focusing the mind and eyes on the space between the eyebrows, often accompanied by specific visualizations, mantras, and breathing patterns

- **Sensory channel** Sight, body and sensation, sound, breath

- **Skill** Concentration

- **Tradition** Yoga

- **Similar practices** Kundalini, Trataka, Mantra, Visualization

FEELING & GAZING

Gazing at your Third Eye from within is the most subtle of the techniques shown here, and the most challenging.

01 Sit in a comfortable posture and close your eyes. Take three deep breaths through your nose. Relax your body with every out-breath.

02 Lick your finger and press it between your eyebrows for a few seconds to sensitize the area.

03 Focus your mind on the Third Eye internally. Spend a few minutes just feeling that area, as if your whole consciousness exists only in that spot.

04 Without opening your eyes, slightly raise them as if you are gazing at the Third Eye from within.

05 Keep your eyes steady, slightly pointing up towards the centre. This helps calm and interiorize the mind. Don't strain or raise the eyes too much.

06 Keep your awareness there, both feeling and gazing at that spot.

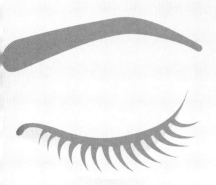

"Let go of thoughts or images that arise, and return your attention to the practice."

VISUALIZATION

If you are more of a visual person, you can use visualization to bring your attention to the Third Eye.

01 Sit in a comfortable posture and close your eyes. Take three deep breaths through your nose. Relax your body with every out-breath.

02 Lick your finger and press it between your eyebrows for a few seconds to sensitize the area.

03 Focus your mind on the Third Eye internally. Spend a few minutes just feeling that area, as if your whole consciousness exists only in that spot.

04 Visualize a small star in front of your eyebrow centre – a bright white dot in the middle of darkness. Or, visualize a shining sun on the horizon.

05 If the image moves about or fades, try to make it stable. If you can't visualize it, simply imagine it is there, or feel its presence.

MANTRA

In this technique you "feel" a pulsation in the Third Eye in sync with a mantra to help focus your attention there.

01 Sit in a comfortable posture and close your eyes. Take three deep breaths through your nose. Relax your body with every out-breath.

02 Lick your finger and press it between your eyebrows for a few seconds to sensitize the area.

03 Focus your mind on the Third Eye internally. Spend a few minutes just feeling that area, as if your whole consciousness exists only in that spot.

04 Try to feel a small pulsation on the spot of your Third Eye. If you still can't feel it after a few minutes, just imagine the feeling of pulsation there.

05 Mentally repeat the mantra "om" while focusing on the Third Eye, in sync with that pulsation.

BREATHING

This meditation technique uses the breath and imagination to channel your focus to the Third Eye.

01 Sit in a comfortable posture and close your eyes. Take three deep breaths through your nose. Relax your body with every out-breath.

02 Lick your finger and press it between your eyebrows for a few seconds to sensitize the area.

03 Focus your mind on the Third Eye internally. Spend a few minutes just feeling that area, as if your whole consciousness exists only in that spot.

04 Focus on your breathing as it moves through the nostrils. Move your consciousness with the breath.

05 As you breathe in, feel the air and your awareness travelling in through your nostrils and up to the Third Eye. Hold it there for a moment.

06 As you breathe out, feel the air and your awareness travelling from the Third Eye through the nostrils.

MANTRA

A lullaby for the mind

A mantra is a word, syllable, or short sentence that is repeated out loud, as a whisper, or simply in your mind. Like the breath, mantras are one of the most widespread tools of meditation, present in many traditions.

WHY CHOOSE THIS PRACTICE?

Mantras are a very effective means of meditation, especially for beginners, as they easily bring a sense of calmness, stability, and homogeneity to your mind. As mantras and thoughts both take the form of words, focusing on a mantra can also help to diminish thinking.

In a spiritual context, mantras are very specific words that denote the Divine in its various forms. For a secular approach, you can choose any word, but it is important that you connect to its meaning and sound. If you don't know which to use, try "om" or "so-ham". These are universal and have a deeply calming effect. Once you choose your mantra, or are given one by your teacher, it is best not to change it.

After you repeat a mantra daily for several months, it can tend to "play itself" in the background of your mind – at this point, the practice becomes more about listening to the mantra.

KEY FACTS

- **Essence** Repeating a sound, word, or phrase as an aid to pacify and transform the mind
- **Sensory channel** Sound
- **Skill** Concentration, awareness
- **Tradition** Yoga, Vedic
- **Similar practices** Kirtan

---

02 Keeping your eyes open, repeat your mantra out loud several times, for about a minute. If your mind is tense, agitated, or lethargic, you might want to spend longer repeating the mantra out loud.

01 Sit in a meditation posture and close your eyes. Take three deep breaths through your nose. Relax your body with every out-breath.

om mmmmmmmmmm

04 Repeat the mantra mentally. Stop moving your lips, tongue, and throat. If your mind becomes too noisy or sleepy, go back to whispering or repeating it out loud. If it helps, keep your eyes half-open, but without gazing at anything. You can also sync your mantra with the breath.

03 Close your eyes and continue repeating your mantra, but as a whisper. Move your lips and tongue, but make the sound so faint that you can barely hear it. If your mind is agitated, repeat the mantra at a faster pace to overpower your thoughts. As your mind calms down and turns inside, the repetition can slow down.

05 Feel the effect of the mantra in your body and mind. Don't let it become mechanical or lifeless, but don't concentrate too hard on it. Let thoughts come, but always keep part of your attention with your mantra.

06 To close, let go of the voluntary repetition of the mantra. If it continues by itself, let it be and just observe it. Then, slowly move your fingers, open your eyes, and finish the practice.

LABELLING

Putting order in the chaos

Labelling, or noting, what we are aware of in our experience – such as thoughts, sensations, or emotions – helps us to be more present and mindful. It is one way to practise Vipassana (see pp.86–87).

WHY CHOOSE THIS PRACTICE?

Labelling is a way of seeing your own thoughts and feelings more objectively, without reacting, which makes it good training for techniques such as Vipassana or Mindfulness. It helps you gain clarity when you have multiple chains of thoughts and feelings simultaneously, or when you have repetitive thoughts, and can help you learn more about yourself.

Labelling can be a standalone practice, but it is also good preparation for other open monitoring meditations, or whenever you feel you need to put some order into the chaos – for example, if there is a lot of confusion in the mind, or when very powerful thoughts or emotions are at play.

KEY FACTS

• **Essence** Placing mental labels on your thoughts and sensations

• **Sensory channel** Mind

• **Skill** Awareness

• **Tradition** Buddhism

• **Similar practices** Mindfulness, Vipassana, Inner Silence, Mini-meditation 4

03 You can repeat the label, to emphasize it – for example, "thinking, thinking" or "hearing, hearing". If a thought or feeling continues, keep repeating the label until it passes.

02 In your mind, start labelling whatever thought, sensation, or emotion is predominant in your consciousness. You can use a generic, single word. For example, if memories arise, label this "remembering", or if it is random thinking, label it "thinking". Other labels could be "pain", "anxiety", "desire", or "frustration". Use whichever word comes to mind first.

01 You can practise this technique in any position, but a seated meditation posture can help deepen the experience.

04 If you are paying attention to your breathing, you can use labels such as "in, in", "breathing in, breathing in", or "rising, rising", and adapt for breathing out.

05 Keep your labelling alive and gentle. It is not a pushing away, and it should not become mechanical. If your mind is really busy, you may wish to label more frequently.

06 Once the mind quietens down, you may want to label less often, or even let go of labelling altogether and simply pay attention to your present moment experience as it is, without words.

07 Finally, if you haven't already, let go of the labelling and just rest in your natural awareness for a few moments. Then, slowly move your body, and open your eyes.

"The purpose of labelling is not precision, but clear, moment-by-moment awareness of your experience."

INNER SILENCE

The Yogic way to mindfulness and self-mastery

Based on ancient Tantric practices and developed by the Bihar School of Yoga, Inner Silence (*Antar Mouna*) focuses first on developing a firm ground of awareness and mindfulness, before introducing concentration and thoughtlessness.

WHY CHOOSE THIS PRACTICE?

This technique is especially useful if you have a very restless mind and are unable to concentrate when using other techniques. It develops the ability to both witness and direct your mind, which calms the mind and puts some order into the chaos. Inner Silence also develops self-awareness, acceptance, and witnessing.

> **KEY FACTS**
>
> - **Essence** Being aware of sounds, sensations, and thoughts, creating thoughts at will, and cultivating the space beyond thought
> - **Sensory channel** Mind, multi-channel
> - **Skill** Awareness, concentration
> - **Tradition** Yoga
> - **Similar practices** Mindfulness, Vipassana, Labelling, Abstract Meditation, Mini-meditation 4

114

"*Resist nothing and cling to nothing. There is no need to interpret anything.*"

01 Sit in a comfortable meditation posture and close your eyes. Take three deep breaths through your nose. Allow your body to relax more with every out-breath.

02 Become aware of the sounds you hear. Let every sound reach your ears as it is. Don't analyze. Don't resist. Don't cling to any sound. Allow your attention to scan all the sounds you can hear, one by one.

03 Become aware of sensations in your body. Notice hot and cold, pressure and lightness, tension and relaxation. Observe them as they are, without interpreting them. No clinging and no resistance. Finally, become aware of your breathing. Notice if it is deep or shallow, fast or slow, through the chest or abdomen.

04 Move your awareness to the mind and its landscape of thoughts, feelings, and images. Watch its every movement as a detached observer. All that arises is an image on the screen of consciousness: you are the screen. Everything is allowed to show up, be it positive or negative. Don't follow any thought, but remain the passive witness of everything.

05 Be aware that you are thinking and move from passive observer to active agent. Select a thought and think only that one. Don't let other thoughts distract you, or branch off into unrelated thoughts: think on purpose, not randomly. After a few moments, dispose of the thought. Do this two more times.

06 A more advanced stage is to focus on the empty space in the mind, the silent background from which all thoughts arise and into which they dissolve. This is consciousness. If thoughts or images arise, leave them aside and keep gazing at this inner space of "no thought".

07 To conclude the meditation, bring your attention back to your body and breathing. After a moment, slowly move your fingers and open your eyes.

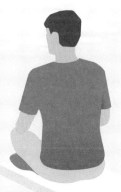

NETI NETI

Not this, not that

Neti Neti is a meditation formula found in the Vedas. It is not religious by nature, but simply invites us to fully realize a simple fact of our experience: that whatever we perceive is not who we are.

WHY CHOOSE THIS PRACTICE?

This meditation seeks to develop clarity about who you are by releasing identification with all that you are not. For example, you know that you are not your shirt. You existed before you bought it and you will exist after you get rid of it. That is why you say "my shirt" – it is separate from you.

As obvious as this seems, we don't apply the same idea to our body, mind, thoughts, and feelings. You say "my body", "my mind", "my thoughts", "my feelings", and you feel that they belong to you, but what is this "you" they belong to? You don't know, but you can be clear about what you are not. For example, you may have a negative thought such as "I am worthless". You are likely to identify with this thought and suffer it, but in reality, this thought is not you.

KEY FACTS

- **Essence** Refusing to identify with anything you can perceive, and remaining as the observer
- **Sensory channel** Mind
- **Skill** Awareness
- **Tradition** Vedic
- **Similar practices** Self-Enquiry, Vipassana, Mini-meditation 4

---

04 Become aware of your whole body. Recognize that it is also an object in your awareness. Repeat the affirmation again, this time about your body and its changing states.

03 Observe all the bodily sensations you perceive. Recognize that they too are objects in your awareness. Repeat the same affirmation, but now about sensations.

01 You can do this meditation in any position, but a seated posture may help you go deeper. Close your eyes and breathe deeply a few times to settle down.

02 Observe the sounds you hear. Recognize that they are objects in your awareness. Tell yourself:

"...I am aware of these sounds, so they are not me and not mine. I am the observing consciousness.**"**

05 Observe your thoughts, whatever they are at this moment. They are like sounds and images flying through the space of your awareness. This time, repeat the affirmation, making your thoughts your focus.

06 Contemplate your feelings, memories, desires, and personality in the same way. Before they arose, you already existed. Once they disappear, you will still remain as you are. You perceive them, so they are objects in your awareness. You are the subject, the perceiver, the observer of them.

07 Your own name, the roles you perform in this world, your identity – contemplate how all these things are not who you are. You are aware of them and you existed before them.

08 Step by step, you release identification with everything else, and gain clarity about your real nature: consciousness. Then, remain as what remains: that is you. It is pure awareness, the witnessing consciousness. Stay here for a few minutes.

09 To close the meditation, bring your attention back to the body for a couple of minutes. Feel your whole body. Feel your breathing pattern. Slowly move your fingers and open your eyes.

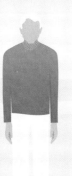

EXPAND YOUR CONSCIOUSNESS

Experiencing the whole cosmos

This meditation is an exercise in imagination, visualization, and feeling. Its purpose is to expand your sense of self beyond the limits of your body and mind, embracing the whole universe. The result is a feeling of liberation.

WHY CHOOSE THIS PRACTICE?
Focusing on something as large as the universe has the effect of quietening the mind and taking you beyond the intellect, making all your problems seem small and insignificant. It also creates a feeling of spaciousness and peace within you and a sense of unity with everything. This is the basis for true empathy, compassion, and connection.

   The stronger your ability to visualize and really feel what you imagine, the better the effects of this practice. However, this technique may not appeal to you if you prefer to be strongly grounded in your body and its sensations.

118

KEY FACTS

● **Essence** Expanding your sense of self to encompass the whole universe

● **Sensory channel** Mind

● **Skill** Awareness

● **Tradition** Many, particularly Tantra Yoga

● **Similar practices** Abstract Meditation, Visualization, Headless Me

04 Expand your awareness to your neighbourhood. It is your new body – every person, building, and living being there is now inside of you.

03 Expand your awareness to the room you are in. Feel that it is your new self. Your consciousness permeates the whole room completely.

02 Bring your awareness to your whole body. Feel it as an entire unit. See your body from the outside, in the eye of your mind: front, back, left, right, above, then from all directions simultaneously.

01 Sit in a comfortable posture and close your eyes. Take three deep breaths through your nose. Your body becomes still and relaxed with every out-breath.

Enjoy this feeling of limitlessness, vastness, lightness, and space.

05 Expand your awareness to your whole city or town. Then your country. Then the planet. Do your problems feel smaller now? Is your sense of self broadened? If thoughts come, just let them go, and return to your visualization.

06 Expand your awareness to include the entire universe. All the billions of planets, stars, galaxies, beings, light, and space – it's all you now. Allow your sense of self to embrace the whole universe.

07 You are infinite. Feel how large and spacious you are. You are beyond all limitation, beyond any individual name or form. And you are the witness of the whole cosmos, the observer of it all. Be still, and relax in this recognition.

08 Slowly bring your attention back to the room. Hear the sounds in your environment, one by one. Become aware of your body, its shape and size. Remember its position inside the room, and the time of the day.

09 Pay attention to your breathing for a few moments. Consciously make your breathing deeper. Slowly move your fingers, hands, shoulders, then open your eyes.

HEADLESS ME

Turning off the thinking mind

We live a lot of our life inside our heads: it's where all our thoughts, memories, frustrations, desires, and problems live. In Headless Me, the aim is to get some distance from our minds by operating more from the heart and the body level.

WHY CHOOSE THIS PRACTICE?

Headless Me comes from the Tantra Yoga tradition, which describes many unusual meditations – some use esoteric concepts, while others, such as the one shown here, use imagination, visualization, or feelings as their object of meditation.

Headless Me is a simple but powerful exercise in imagination. It may feel a little macabre for some, but others will find it incredibly liberating. The key is to let your imagination flow freely and really feel as if you don't have a head. You can also do this with your eyes open, standing in front of a mirror. However, this meditation is not advised for those suffering from derealization, depersonalization, or dissociative identity disorders.

> **KEY FACTS**
>
> - **Essence** Imagine you have no head and enjoy the space
> - **Sensory channel** Mind
> - **Skill** Concentration
> - **Tradition** Yoga
> - **Similar practices** Meditations from the Tantras, Zazen, Visualization

01 Close your eyes and breathe deeply, settling down in the present moment.

02 Take a couple of minutes to mentally scan your whole body, from head to toes: left leg and foot, right leg and foot, belly and chest, the whole back, left arm and hand, right arm and hand, shoulders and neck, head and face. Develop awareness of your whole body. Hold it in your consciousness as a single unit.

03 Imagine that you have no head. Everything is fine with you. You feel present, peaceful, and well. The only thing that is different is that your body ends above your shoulders. After that, where the neck and head would be, there is only space.

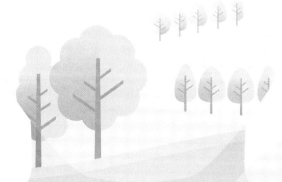

"The sky is your head: feel that space."

07 Slowly start moving your body, open your eyes, and conclude the meditation.

06 When you're ready, visualize your head coming back into place above your body, but internally hold on to that feeling of spaciousness, presence, and openness.

05 Visualize yourself without a head. Really feel as if this is true. See yourself going about your day, getting everything done, but without a head. Nobody is noticing that you have no head, but you have an amazing feeling of peace, silence. Where is your centre? Your "self"? Do you miss it? Spend as much time as you like enjoying this space.

04 Thoughts have nowhere to come from and nowhere to land. It's all spacious and boundless. All your thoughts, your ego, your personality, and complications are gone. In its place there is only space: empty, vast, open.

ABSTRACT MEDITATION

Thinking the unthinkable

Many meditation traditions – including Tibetan Buddhism and Jnana Yoga – include abstract forms of meditation. In all of them, the focus is on expansive concepts that take you beyond the limitations of the ego.

WHY CHOOSE THIS PRACTICE?

Abstract meditation is based on the idea that the mind develops the qualities of whatever it keeps thinking about. So, if you think about things that annoy or scare you, your mind becomes restless and miserable, whereas contemplating space or infinity will make your mind vast and open.

Ultimately, the goal is to give the mind a thought it likes to hold on to that is expansive by nature, such as infinity, eternity, universal love, God, space, time, or consciousness. Try any you feel attracted to, but once you have settled on a concept, work with only that one for some time. Reading a short passage about it before meditation can help, but if this makes your mind discursive and busy, there is no need. Finally, bring your concept to mind for a few moments during your day to keep it alive and allow you to go deeper into it when you next meditate.

KEY FACTS

- **Essence** Contemplating an abstract concept
- **Sensory channel** Mind
- **Skill** Concentration
- **Tradition** Many
- **Similar practices** Zazen, Expand Your Consciousness, Self-Enquiry

02 Concentrate all your attention on your chosen concept. Contemplate it deeply. Let it permeate your whole mind. Try to feel its meaning, as if it is a reality under your skin.

03 Don't branch off into discursive thinking or association with other thoughts. Just hold on to your concept and dive deep into its essence.

01 You can do this meditation in any position, but a seated posture may help you to meditate more deeply. Close your eyes and breathe deeply a few times, settling in to the present moment.

"The goal is to have a direct, wordless experience of the reality behind your chosen concept."

05 When you are ready, bring your attention back to your body for a few minutes. Feel your whole body and your breathing pattern. Slowly move your fingers and toes, then open your eyes.

04 If your mind gets distracted, repeat the name of your concept in your mind a few times to bring your attention back to contemplation. For example: "infinity, infinity, infinity".

SELF-ENQUIRY

Who am I?

Self-Enquiry (*atma-vichara*) uses the question "Who am I?" to isolate the "I am" from the thoughts and limitations that are usually added to it, and attain the subjective feeling of pure existence, or "I am".

WHY CHOOSE THIS PRACTICE?

"I am" is usually connected to our thoughts and identifications, such as "I am feeling anxious" or "I am a teacher", all of which show the limited ego or personality. The essential part is the "I am" – this is the constant element, the real you. The "I am" knows no suffering. It is simply an expansive sense of being.

Most practices ask you to concentrate or observe, so the subject (the "I" or "I am") focuses on an object, such as the breath. Self-Enquiry, however, is a non-dual meditation: the subject focuses on itself, in other words, it is being itself, without an object.

KEY FACTS

- **Essence** Turning your attention from the seen to the seer
- **Sensory channel** Mind
- **Skill** Concentration, awareness
- **Tradition** Vedic, specifically the Advaita Vedanta tradition
- **Similar practices** Neti Neti

03 Every time you ask these questions, the thought might come, "It is me!" Then ask, "Who am I?" or "What is this I?"

02 Notice the sounds you hear. Ask yourself: "Who am I that hears these sounds?" Notice the sensations you feel. Ask yourself: "Who am I that feels these sensations?" Notice the thoughts you perceive. Ask yourself: "Who am I that perceives these thoughts?" Notice your experience as a whole. Ask yourself: "Who is the one experiencing this?"

01 Sit in a comfortable posture and close your eyes. Take three deep breaths through your nose. Allow your body to become still and relaxed with every out-breath.

"*I am this, I am that is where suffering lives: it is the fake self, limited by these additions.*"

04 Reject any answers that come, as they are also thoughts, which are perceived by you. The answer to this question is not a thought.

05 Move your attention away from what you perceive, back to the perceiver. The perceiver is a space of pure awareness, pure being.

06 Once you find the feeling of pure "I am", stabilize your attention in that space. Focus on the "I am". Relax inside "I am", and let go of all else. Hold on to that wordless sense or presence, and don't try to define it.

07 Whenever your attention gets engaged in thoughts or anything else that you perceive, use the question "Who am I that perceives this?" to bring your attention back to the pure "I am".

08 To conclude, bring your attention back to your whole body. Observe your breathing for a few moments, then slowly open your eyes and move out of the meditation posture.

ZUOWANG

Sitting and forgetting

Based on the Taoist concept of *wu wei* (non-action), Zuowang means "sitting in oblivion". It asks you to switch off the mind, forget body and environment, and enter a space of inexplicable silence.

WHY CHOOSE THIS PRACTICE?

Zuowang is a challenging but direct practice that takes you to a place of no-mind, stillness, and spacious awareness. It is based on the understanding that the normal way that our minds function is artificial, dualistic, and distorted. By allowing the mind to quiet down you are able to dissolve the sense of self and rest in the Tao. There are no concrete instructions for Zuowang, but the steps shown here can help you develop the right attitude for this practice.

KEY FACTS

- **Essence** Letting go of everything and resting in an effortless state of no-mind

- **Sensory channel** Mind

- **Skill** Awareness

- **Tradition** Taoism

- **Similar practices** Zazen, Self-Enquiry, Meditations from the Tantras

03 Whatever is arising in your awareness is empty. It is not your enemy and need not be rejected. Everything is allowed to arise and to be whatever it is – it is all part of the experience. The difference is that, internally, you are in a state of non-doing.

02 Have the attitude of letting go of everything. Forget your surroundings, as if the dimmer switch of your senses has been turned down. Your body is motionless. No sensations are registering. Forget your body. You have no beginning or end. No anchor, support, or form. Forget all concepts or beliefs. Hold no frame of reference, no map of reality.

01 Sit in a meditation posture, straight and unsupported. This helps to stabilize your mind and energy. Your breathing should be smooth, slow, and natural. Close your eyes.

05 Constantly release any tendency of the mind to think about things, to try to understand things, or want to change things. Let it all slip away effortlessly. Allow the conceptual mind to lose all its supports, and become empty on its own.

06 Simply sit in silence, doing nothing in particular, but resting in open and choiceless awareness. Let everything else drop away from you. Release the disturbance of likes and dislikes, of trying, and of knowing. Release the disturbance of a personal identity.

04 Don't start any activity. Don't engage with anything that is perceived. Hold no preference towards anything that arises. Hold no intention to do anything, or to control or change anything.

07 Don't try to "do" nothing. Release all trying and non-trying. Just be here and now, present but empty of everything. Remain present, and let the cultivation of this state happen naturally. By itself, the mind will become quiet and you will feel grounded and one.

08 Immerse yourself in the unfathomable emptiness of the universe. Allow your being to permeate everything. This is your original nature, open and wide, without any self-referencing.

09 When you are ready, bring your attention back to your body and breathing. Slowly move your fingers and head, then open your eyes.

"Zuowang is like the open sky, above all clouds: so vast that you aren't even aware of the clouds."

MEDITATIONS FROM THE TANTRAS

The discovery of emptiness

Adapted from contemplations in the Vijnanabhairava Tantra, an ancient text that describes 112 techniques, these meditations involve creative contemplations and visualizations.

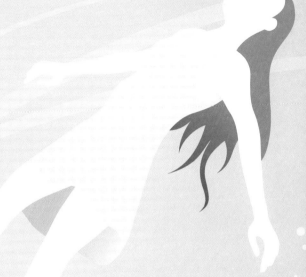

WHY CHOOSE THIS PRACTICE?

From the spiritual perspective of Tantra, the purpose of these meditations is to see all things as manifestations of consciousness, overcome the ego, and merge the individual mind in the universal mind. Practised in a secular way, they serve to free you from slavery to emotions, desires, and sensations, and help you to develop self-knowledge and cultivate empathy by contemplating the oneness of all things. Those shown here are are grouped by their focus on the body, mind, or senses. Try any you feel an attraction towards.

KEY FACTS

• **Essence** A group of unusual practices that free the mind from attachment and realize the emptiness and oneness of all things

• **Sensory channel** Mind, body and sensation, sound

• **Skill** Concentration, awareness

• **Tradition** Yoga, specifically Tantra

• **Similar practices** Visualization, Headless Me, Abstract Meditation, Expand Your Consciousness

"*Discover new ways to access a state of stillness, silence, and inner freedom.*"

BODY TECHNIQUES

These meditations invite you to concentrate on your body in imaginative ways to change the state of your mind and your sense of self. For many of us, our attention readily connects to the body as a basic frame of reference, so here, Tantra asks you to start from where you are.

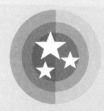

FLOATING IN SPACE

Concentrating on the feeling of weightlessness enables the mind to become light and thoughtless.

01 For this technique, it is best to sit on a comfortable chair or sofa.

02 Focus all your attention only on your body.

03 Feel as if your body has no support. It is as if floating in space, completely weightless – a zero-gravity experience. Focus on that feeling with full conviction.

04 Concentrate on this feeling of having no support. Use this as the object of your meditation.

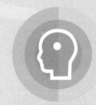

INSIDE THE SKULL

Focusing all your awareness on one tiny spot, your mind becomes quiet and still.

01 Sit in a meditation posture. Close your eyes and take three deep breaths through your nose. Let your body relax with every out-breath.

02 Spend a minute centring your attention in your body. Allow the mind to settle down with the body.

03 Focus all your attention inside your skull. Imagine that you are a tiny sphere of light existing in the middle of the darkness of your skull.

04 Focus all your being in that small spot, completely still. If thoughts or images appear, let them be and let them pass. Remain still in that spot.

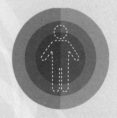

AN EMPTY SHELL

Contemplating the complete emptiness of the body opens up a sense of spaciousness within you.

01 Sit in a meditation posture. Close your eyes and take three deep breaths through your nose. Let your body relax with every out-breath.

02 Spend a minute centring your attention in your body. Allow the mind to settle down with the body.

03 Imagine your body being completely empty – your skin is like an outer shell with nothing inside.

04 If your body is empty and insubstantial, then who are you? You are awareness, inside and out, without being limited to the body.

05 Remain as that sense of pure awareness, of spaciousness, while contemplating the emptiness of the body.

CONTINUED ▶

SENSE TECHNIQUES

Each of these techniques uses a different sense or sensation to focus your attention. By using feelings – such as pleasure or pain – as the object of your meditation, you experience them in their totality, gain insight about their nature, and are able to transcend them.

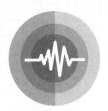

FROM SOUND TO SILENCE

In this technique, you focus on the sound of a chant, but you could use a singing bowl or an instrument. You will need a very quiet setting.

01 Sit in a meditation posture. Close your eyes and take three deep breaths through your nose. Let your body relax with every out-breath.

02 Spend a minute centring your attention in your body. Allow the mind to settle down with the body.

03 Chant the mantra "om", stretching the "mmm" sound a lot. Pay attention to the whole length of the sound, starting strong and becoming quieter until it vanishes.

04 Just as the sound rises from silence and dissolves back to silence, allow it to guide your awareness back into silence.

05 Once the sound has gone, keep paying attention to the silence. After a few moments, chant "om" again and repeat the process as many times as you like.

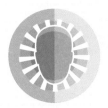

ORGASMIC MEDITATION

Here, you focus on the feeling of joy, and learn to transcend it so you can access it whenever you like.

01 Sit in a meditation posture. Close your eyes and take three deep breaths through your nose. Let your body relax with every out-breath.

02 Spend a minute centring your attention in your body. Allow the mind to settle down with the body.

03 Remember a time when you felt a deep sense of joy, pleasure, or satisfaction, like eating delicious food.

04 Expand this feeling by becoming deeply aware of it. Focus on it. Let your mind become one with it. Lose yourself in it, but keep your awareness open and clear.

05 Transcend the joy by making it so intense that it takes you beyond yourself, to the joy of pure consciousness. Trace the feeling back to its source in your consciousness. The memory of it is just a trigger to access this inner pool of joy anytime.

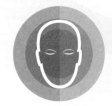

PEACE BEYOND PAIN

This meditation uses physical pain as an object of meditation, and teaches you to accept it without aversion.

01 Sit in a meditation posture. Close your eyes and take three deep breaths through your nose. Let your body relax with every out-breath.

02 Spend a minute centring your attention in your body. Allow the mind to settle down with the body.

03 It is hard to ignore pain and easy to focus on it, so take it as an object of your meditation. Keep all your awareness in the place in your body where the pain is felt most acutely.

04 Observe the sensation of pain, and surrender. Let go of any aversion towards the pain. Relax inside of it and become comfortable with it.

05 Go beyond the surface and simply accept that sensation as a sensation, without labelling it as good or bad, pleasant or unpleasant. Let your mind rest in the quiet and open witnessing of this sensation in its pure expression.

"You can learn to access feelings of intense bliss or joy any time you like."

CONTINUED ▶

"You can find space between your thoughts, like the pause between music notes."

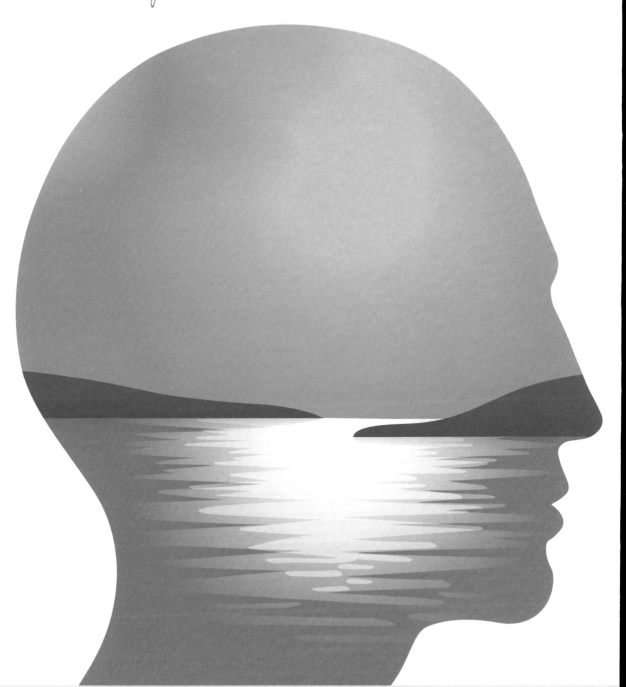

MIND TECHNIQUES

The creative contemplations and visualizations shown here challenge you to find stillness, freedom, and expansiveness in your mind, and broaden your sense of self to include everyone.

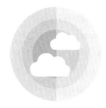

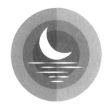

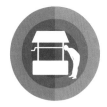

THE SPACE BETWEEN THOUGHTS

Learn to focus on the space between your thoughts, so you can always rest part of your awareness there.

01 Sit in a meditation posture. Close your eyes and take three deep breaths through your nose. Let your body relax with every out-breath.

02 Spend a minute centring your attention in your body. Allow the mind to settle down with the body.

03 Look inside your mind and observe whatever thoughts are there. Try to focus on the space between one thought and the next, like the pause between notes in music, however fast the rhythm might be. This can be extremely difficult in the beginning because our awareness is not trained to be so sharp. But if you look intently and persevere, it is possible.

04 Before any thought arises, and after it is gone, there is space and silence. The more you train yourself to notice and dwell in this space, the larger the gaps between your thoughts will become.

ONE SELF

This technique moves beyond the self by asking you to contemplate the oneness of all life and consciousness.

01 Sit in a meditation posture. Close your eyes and take three deep breaths through your nose. Let your body relax with every out-breath.

02 Spend a minute centring your attention in your body. Allow the mind to settle down with the body.

03 Forget about your body and mind, and contemplate that inside every person there is only one self. The same consciousness is shining as "I" behind every mind.

04 Just as the moon appears as many different reflections in different pools of water, the same consciousness appears differently through many minds.

BOTTOMLESS WELL

Here, your mind moves freely as there is nothing to obstruct it. You can also try staring into a real well.

01 Sit in a meditation posture. Close your eyes and take three deep breaths through your nose. Let your body relax with every out-breath.

02 Spend a minute centring your attention in your body. Allow the mind to settle down with the body.

03 Imagine sitting in front of a bottomless well. You look down it, but your sight meets no objects, so there is nothing to think about.

04 Allow your mind to continuously delve into this bottomless well. Your mind lets go of all other supports, and moves freely without resistance.

05 Focus all your attention on this sense of infinite expansion and going deep without end.

LOVING-KINDNESS MEDITATION

Purification of the heart

Loving-Kindness, or *metta* in Pali, is one of the four "divine abodes" or "sublime attitudes" that Buddhists seek to develop. In this practice, you generate the feelings of love and benevolence, and wish happiness and wellbeing on yourself and others.

WHY CHOOSE THIS PRACTICE?

Loving-Kindness Meditation helps you to cultivate positive emotions and to let go of negative emotions such as anger, hatred, indifference, selfishness, ill-will, and sadness (see also pp.24–25). Once kindled, you focus on the feeling of Loving-Kindness as the object of your concentration, which makes it grow even more. When that happens, you'll have feelings of joy, openness, and bliss in your heart.

134

02 Try to remember a time when you felt deeply accepted, loved, and appreciated for who you are. If it's helpful, remember who made you feel that way and the events around it. If you can't think of a specific example, imagine how it would feel. Create an image in your mind, as if it's a film, and experience those feelings.

01 Sit in a meditation posture and close your eyes. Take three deep breaths through your nose. Relax your body with every out-breath.

KEY FACTS

- **Essence** Kindling and growing the feeling of Loving-Kindness for yourself and others through memory, visualization, and affirmations

- **Sensory channel** Heart

- **Skill** Concentration

- **Tradition** Buddhism

- **Similar practices** Visualization, Kirtan

03 Once you have kindled the feeling, move your focus to it. Leave behind the details of the memory or image, and just become aware of the feeling. How does it feel in your body, mind, and heart? Take it as the object of your concentration. Keep feeding it, reproducing it, increasing it. If thoughts distract you, recognize that, and return to the feeling.

04 When the feeling is stable, project it towards yourself, towards another person, or towards the whole planet. It can be helpful to visualize the person you are projecting it to (even if it is yourself). Then, with feeling and intention, repeat internally:

"...May you be happy. May you be safe. May you be at peace!"

05 Bring your attention back to your breathing. Observe it for a moment or two. Then become aware of your whole body and its contact with the floor or chair. When you are ready, slowly move your fingers, open your eyes, and conclude the practice.

"When visualizing another person, it is helpful to try to put yourself in their shoes. Imagine that you are them."

SUFI HEARTBEAT MEDITATION

The pulse of the spirit

Sufis, the mystics of Islam, use breathing, meditation, and prayer to achieve union with the Divine. The technique shown here focuses on the heartbeat as a way to gain this connection, but you can perform a secular variation.

WHY CHOOSE THIS PRACTICE?

Sufism is about falling in love with the Divine, or Spirit, and keeping your mind and heart bathing in that blissful feeling of love and surrender. Sufi Heartbeat Meditation is a way to connect to this sense of a greater "spirit" or "intelligence" in life and feel its presence in you. As people seek more experiential and personal ways to connect with a higher power, this technique is becoming increasingly popular.

Though spiritual by nature, you can practise a secular version by simply concentrating on your heartbeat by itself, without repeating any mantra or thinking about God.

KEY FACTS

- **Essence** Focusing on your heartbeat to connect with the Divine
- **Sensory channel** Heart
- **Skill** Awareness
- **Tradition** Sufism
- **Similar practices** Kirtan

01 Sit in a comfortable posture or lie down. Close your eyes and take three deep breaths through your nose. Let your body become relaxed and still with every out-breath.

02 Develop full body awareness by spending a couple of minutes centring your attention in your body. Allow the mind to settle down with the body.

03 Once your body and breathing are calm, start noticing your heartbeat. Focus all your awareness in the centre of your chest, and forget about everything else.

"Your heartbeat is your life. It is the pulsation of life within you."

06 Forget about your body, your thoughts, and yourself. Become a witness to the pulsation of your heart. If your mind wanders, bring it back to your heartbeat. Spend as much time in this phase as you like. If you're practising a secular version, you can now move straight to the final step.

05 Allow your mind and heartbeat to merge together, and the heartbeat to become the rhythm of your whole being, as if there is nothing else. Let all your thoughts be consumed by the heartbeat.

04 Pay attention to every heartbeat, as if you can't miss a single one. If you can't feel your heartbeat, make sure you relax your body fully, quieten the mind, and keep your awareness on the area of the heart. Eventually you will feel it.

07 Awaken the feeling of love and sacredness in the heart by thinking of the Divine or Spirit, in whatever form that takes for you. Or develop love towards life and the Spirit itself. Have a feeling of gratitude, love, and surrender to the larger life of which you are a part.

08 Contemplate your heartbeat as the heartbeat of the Divine, of life itself. Feel the warmth, peace, and sweetness that come with loving the Divine through your heartbeat.

10 To conclude, let go of your heartbeat, and bring your attention to your body as a whole. Develop whole body awareness. Then, when you are ready, slowly move your body, and open your eyes.

09 Alternatively, or in addition to the previous step, repeat a mantra in sync with your heartbeat. The Sufis repeat "Allah", but you can use any mantra while cultivating a sense of love and surrender. If you're not sure, use "om".

INTEGRATING AND DEEPENING

MEDITATIVE MOMENTS

Meditation in daily life

To get the most out of your meditation practice, it should become part of your whole life, rather than a task you "do". Building moments of meditation into your day and adding a meditative quality to your activities will also advance your practice more quickly.

Your meditation affects your daily life, but your daily life also affects your meditation: ideally, they need to support each other. To do this, you can use meditation techniques to take a minute to pause, slow down, and collect your thoughts a few times every day. This could be 5–10 slow, mindful breaths, relaxing any tensions in your body, or bringing your meditation object to mind for a few moments.

You'll need to find a way of remembering to do this: you could use an alarm or notification on your phone or wearable device, a mindfulness reminders app, or a sticky note on your computer monitor.

Ideally, aim to take one pause every two hours. If that sounds like a lot, remember that it's only 60 seconds: the results can feel magical. If that isn't practical, start with just two or three pauses a day.

MAKING YOUR ACTIVITIES MEDITATIVE
You can also cultivate awareness, focus, and relaxation – three of the essential elements of meditation – during your daily activities. Try building some of these eight "meditative moments" into your day.

01 When stopped at a traffic light take a deep breath and relax the muscles in your face, shoulders, and hands.

02 When you're on a train or bus, notice all the information coming through your senses – what you see, hear, and feel.

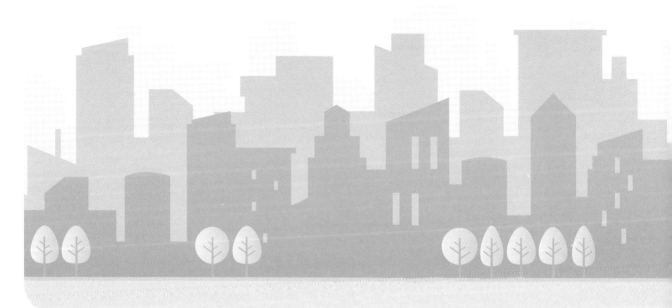

Meditation can enrich your whole life, and your whole life can be training for meditation, if you approach it the right way.

03 Before meeting a difficult person, or facing a difficult situation, take a deep breath and release all negative emotion while exhaling.

04 Treat any task as an exercise of concentration and be fully focused. With any distractions that arise, gently bring your focus back to the task at hand, just as you do with your thoughts when you meditate.

05 Notice the state of your mind while you are using your phone or answering an email. Are you stressed and anxious? Or calm and confident? Whatever it is, try approaching that emotion meditatively (see pp.144–145).

06 Pay attention to the sensations in your body as you eat. Take time to really experience your food: notice its texture and colours. What does it smell like? As you take each mouthful, notice as many flavours as you can. Observe how your mind and body react to each taste.

07 When you unlock your phone with a specific purpose in mind, complete that purpose before you open any other app or notification.

08 When having a conversation with someone, be 100 per cent present: hold their gaze and notice their body language. Really listen to what they are saying, and consider your response.

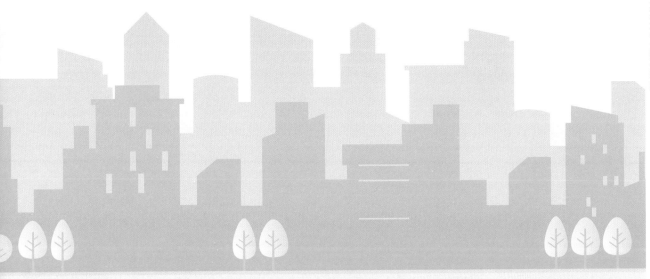

DIGITAL DISTRACTION

How meditation can help

Technology is a wonderful tool, but our increasing interconnectedness can encourage unawareness, restlessness, over-stimulation, and absence from life. Meditation helps us enjoy its benefits while avoiding the pitfalls.

Whatever we seek from technology – whether it's to expand knowledge or to connect with others – it's easy to get drawn into distraction and lose sight of why we use it. And with emails, social media, and text messages constantly pulling our attention towards a screen, it can be particularly challenging to concentrate and find stillness.

This is another reason why the skills we learn through meditation are so important: those who are focused can shut off distractions, say "no" to the temptation of instant gratification, and concentrate on something meaningful, giving them a significantly better chance of succeeding in life. Equally, being aware of how we interact with technology helps us reclaim our power over it, rather than be overpowered by it.

Having a healthier relationship with technology will also help build meditative principles – such as freedom and non-reactivity – into your daily life, which will, in turn, deepen your practice.

PRACTISE SELF-AWARENESS
Being aware of what you seek from technology, and how it affects you, will help you make more conscious choices about how and when you use it. Next time you reach for your phone or computer, become aware of what is moving you to take that action, and notice if you get dragged in a different direction as you interact with your device.

Observe how it feels in your body and mind when you are using technology, before, during, and after. Notice its effects on you: the sensations,

emotions, and thoughts that get triggered. Do you feel relieved when you have read a message, or more anxious? Perhaps you feel a dizzying rush of gratification, followed by a dip of boredom?

REPLACE MINDLESS FOR MINDFUL
For many of us, our natural tendency is to check our smartphones whenever we have an idle minute – from waiting for the bus, to eating our breakfast. Many of us check our phones just before we go to bed and again as soon as we wake up.

Using self-awareness, start noticing when you reach for your phone when there is no real need. Then, try replacing this mindless habit with a mindful one, such as taking a couple of deep breaths, observing your mind, or simply enjoying life happening around you. You could even do a mini-meditation (see pp.44–53). It won't be easy at first, but it will be well worth it.

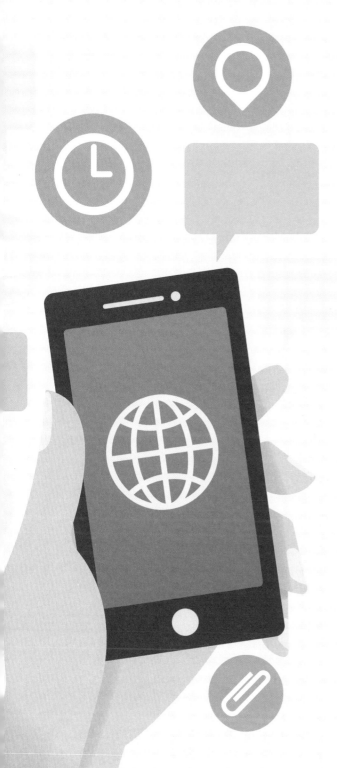

"With technology comes an endless stream of distraction – which is why we need meditation more than ever."

SET SOME GROUND RULES

Once you have developed awareness about your relationship with technology, it's time to take your power back by creating guidelines for how you want use it. Some ideas are:

DON'T USE the Internet before breakfast or after 10pm.

CHECK YOUR EMAILS and social media only 2–3 times a day.

HAVE A SCREEN-FREE day once a week, or once a month.

TAKE ONE LONG BREATH before engaging with any call, email, or message. This is a way to practise the meditative principle of non-reactivity (see pp.144–145).

AIM TO HAVE no more than five apps on your smartphone, tablet, and computer that can send you notifications. If this creates a fear of missing out, simply recognize this feeling, and proceed. If it continues, use meditation to manage that emotion (see pp.144–145).

As with establishing any new habit, following your guidelines will take some willpower – one of the skills you develop in meditation (see p.22).

143

PAUSE, BREATHE, PROCEED

Meditation to manage emotions

Our emotions are involuntary responses to situations, so they can feel out of our control. Meditation gives us the tools to deal with our emotions head-on and teaches us to be less reactive. As a result, we are able to live by design, not default.

How often do you find yourself making a silly mistake, or reacting emotionally to something only to regret it immediately afterwards? This results from living in automatic mode, our default setting, which comes with many costs: shame, bad decisions, and lost opportunities.

We might not always know the best thing to do in every situation, but more often than not we know exactly what we should or shouldn't have done – we just didn't have enough time, in real life, to figure things out and act from a better place. Emotions have an important part to play in this too: we can't stop them from coming up, but we can change how we react to them. With the skills we learn through meditation, we can save ourselves a lot of suffering.

AWARENESS, RELAXATION, FOCUS
By developing greater awareness, meditation helps you become conscious of your emotional states and feelings. This enables you to observe emotions as they are, without judgment and without creating unnecessary stories about them in your mind. You also start to notice your behaviour more, and recognize when your triggers are being fired, not only when the damage is already done.

Relaxing the body and mind in meditation gives you a sense of calm that you can carry into life outside your practice, while keeping your attention on your meditation object sharpens your powers of focus. As a result, situations that would cause you to jump to conclusions, or to say and do things out of reflex, are now less likely to do so, and you are able to notice when your mind drifts into negative patterns of thought or feeling. You can also use these three skills to help uncomfortable or unhelpful emotions subside, or to heighten positive emotions (see opposite).

THE MANTRA OF NON-REACTIVITY
Together, these skills give you less reactivity and more pause, or "non-reactivity", in day-to-day life. When faced with a trigger, this pause is usually enough for your fight-or-flight response to cool down and for your rational brain to kick in, giving you more options for how to react. To deal with powerful emotions, you can also follow the steps on the opposite page.

"Meditation gives you the tools to navigate your emotional world."

HOW TO HANDLE EMOTIONS

By giving you greater awareness of your emotional states and feelings and the skills you need to manage them, meditation equips you to take back control. The first step is to determine what you want to do with the emotion or feeling.

EMOTION

LET IT BE?

Observe what is happening in your body and mind. Don't judge yourself for it, or interpret what is happening. Simply let the emotion play itself out and learn from it. However, it is important not to focus your attention too fully on the emotion, otherwise you can risk "losing yourself" in the process.

CALM IT?

Label the emotion with a single word, such as "anger", "frustration", "sadness", or "insecurity". This will help you to gain clarity and objectivity about what exactly you are feeling, which takes away some of the immediate power of the emotion and makes it more manageable.

HEIGHTEN IT?

Feed the emotion with your undivided attention, just as you increase the feeling of love in Loving-Kindness Meditation by focusing on it (see pp.134–135). Of course, it will eventually pass, as all feelings are impermanent, but this will make it last longer and leave a deeper impression on your mind.

Take 3–5 slow, deep breaths. Try breathing in for 4 seconds, then out for 4 seconds. If you can, do this a few more times with longer breaths. Each emotional state is linked to a pattern of breathing, so changing it can send a signal to your body that helps the emotion subside.

Identify where the emotion is happening in your body – such as tension in the shoulders or pressure in the chest – and consciously release it with every out-breath.

TO CONQUER, VISUALIZE

Meditation to overcome personal challenges

Whatever inner obstacle or personal challenge you face – whether it's a lack of motivation for a project or a lack of confidence before a date – the visualization skills you develop in meditation are a powerful way to help you overcome it.

We all face challenges in our emotional or psychological lives: perhaps it's social anxiety, a tendency to procrastinate, or even a specific kind of negative self-talk that you want to tackle. By improving your ability to visualize, many meditation techniques give you an effective way to succeed in any area you choose.

A TRIAL RUN

Think of your visualization as practice for a time when you will face your personal challenge: you see yourself in that situation, then visualize yourself acting as you want to act, or feeling what you want to feel. The crucial thing here is that you are not visualizing the end goal straight away. If you want to overcome social anxiety, for example, you don't tell yourself that you won't feel anxiety in a particular situation, because if you do feel anxiety in real life, you will think that your visualization hasn't worked. Instead, you visualize the anxiety coming up and you see yourself overcoming it, as shown in the exercise opposite. This means that when you do face anxiety, you will think: "I know how to deal with this. I've overcome this before, so I can do it again!"

The better you are able to visualize, the sooner you will overcome your personal challenges. To strengthen this ability, choose techniques that include visualizations, such as Neiguan (pp.98–99) and Visualization (pp.104–105) or that focus on the sensory channel of sight, such as Trataka (pp.102–103) or Third Eye Meditations 1 and 2 (pp.108–109).

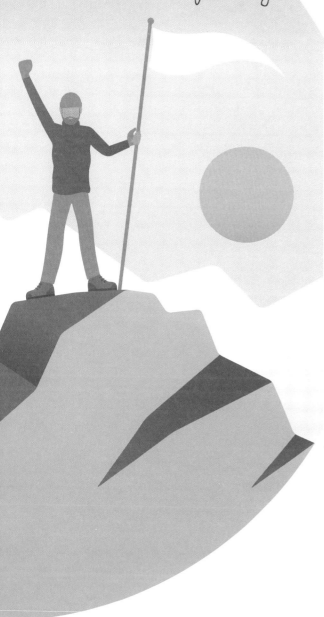

"Visualization is a powerful tool in changing your mindset, feelings, and behaviour."

FOCUS ON CONQUERING SOCIAL ANXIETY

This technique uses visualization to help you prepare for an event that may cause social anxiety, but you can adapt it for any personal challenge.

01 Sit or lie down comfortably. Close your eyes and take a few deep breaths through your nose. Let your body relax and your mind settle down.

02 Visualize the situation that may trigger social anxiety in you. It could be a networking event or a date. Imagine yourself in that situation. See it vividly, adding as much detail as you can.

03 Really see yourself there. Feel how it would feel in your body. Observe the thoughts that would be triggered. Do whatever you need to make the anxiety show up as though it is really happening.

04 See yourself becoming aware that you are anxious, remembering to breathe deeply. Visualize yourself taking a few deep breaths and relaxing your body. See that after a few moments the anxiety is gone. You feel calm and present.

05 Visualize yourself acting with confidence: perhaps speaking assertively, or introducing yourself with a firm handshake. If you can, spend about 5–10 minutes doing this. Allow it to be very real and leave a strong impression on your mind. You can also use affirmations to support this state.

06 When you are ready, let the visualization go. Observe your breathing for a few moments and say to yourself: "I know how to deal with social anxiety. I can overcome it every time."

TO CONQUER, VISUALIZE

POWER YOUR PROBLEM-SOLVING MIND

Meditation for mental clarity

Think how much better you'd be able to solve life's problems if you could boost your focus and clarity, reduce mental noise, and see the bigger picture. Fortunately, these are all skills that meditation can give you.

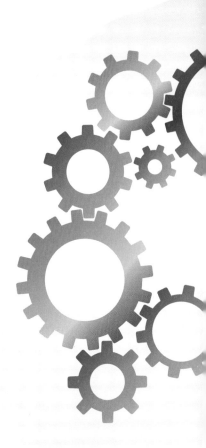

When you're thinking about a problem you need to solve, such as a technical difficulty at work or an issue in your personal life, it's likely that you'll have several other chains of thought moving through your mind, all competing with your thought about the problem. Meditation helps diminish this noise and distraction, and give more focus where it's needed.

ATTENTION AND FOCUS

Meditation trains you to continuously zoom your attention in on your meditation object, and the more attention you give to your object, the clearer it becomes in your awareness. This continuity and stability of attention improves your clarity of thought, which is closely related to your powers of focus.

After a few months of daily training, and with a stronger power of focus, the problem you are trying to solve may only need to compete with one extra chain of thought. This frees up a lot of cognitive power to focus on the task at hand. Many meditators also find that zooming out of their thoughts and into awareness helps them see the bigger picture.

Try meditating for 5–10 minutes before tackling a problem so that you can start with a clean slate. Techniques that are more body- or senses-based, rather than mind- or feelings-based, help give you more space from the problem. For really difficult issues, try the exercise on the opposite page instead.

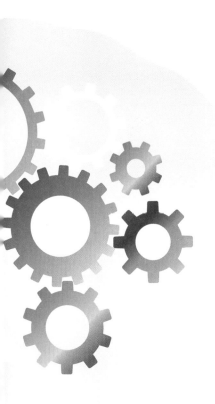

"With focus, clarity, and perspective, you'll be able to solve your problems creatively."

FOCUS ON SOLVING PROBLEMS

Follow this exercise without expectation. You may find that your answers come later, or during your meditation practice the following day, when you have completely forgotten about it.

01 Spend 10–15 minutes thinking about your subject, taking note of all its variables. You could use a big sheet of paper or a whiteboard. Let your thinking be wide, not deep: it's about seeing all the variables and how they relate to each other.

02 Meditate for 20 minutes, ideally with a concentration type of meditation focused on the body or senses. As much as you can, forget all about your subject. This gives space for your subconscious mind to absorb and process all the information it has just received.

03 Just before you finish your meditation, let go of the meditation object and bring your problem back to your mind. Make that problem, in its entirety, the object of your meditation.

04 Don't actively think about your problem. Just let those ideas come up in your awareness by briefly reviewing all the variables of your problem. Remain open, with panoramic awareness, simply watching those ideas play in your mind. See if you discover any new insights or relationships.

05 Conclude your meditation and return to your sheet of paper or whiteboard. You will be in a much better condition to solve your problem creatively and effectively.

Cognitive power
By developing your focus skills and reducing mental noise, meditation frees up more cognitive power to solve problems.

GROW AND FLOURISH

Developing personal strengths through meditation

We already know that meditation helps us to develop important personal strengths such as calmness, patience, and focus, but it also gives us the tools to make long-term changes in any area we choose, from developing courage to kindness.

Long-term personal growth, such as developing a personal strength, requires self-awareness and willpower – two core skills that you enhance through meditation. First, you need self-awareness to recognize opportunities to practise that personal strength, then you need willpower to bring your attention to your chosen way of interacting with the world and follow through with it. You train to do this in meditation many times: noticing that your mind is distracted, and then bringing your attention back to where you want it to be.

Although meditation gives you these two skills, the transformation is not automatic: you still need to make active use of them and do the work needed, outside of meditation.

STARTING WITH THE BODY

Before you change what's happening in your mind, it can help to use the self-awareness you develop through techniques such as Yoga Nidra (see pp.92–93), Vipassana (see pp.86–87), and Mindfulness Meditation (see pp.82–83) to trigger the physical states that usually come with whatever virtue you want to develop. For example, if you are seeking to develop the virtue of courage, try to identify how it feels in your body when you lack courage, or back down from something. Perhaps this is a tension in your shoulders and a churning in your stomach. Then, do the same to imagine how it feels once you have used courage to overcome a fear or anxiety. You might remember a time where you felt courageous, and took action regardless of fear, or use your imagination to feel what that would be like. This could be a sense of expansion in your chest and energy in your muscles. Understanding this difference will enable you to create the quality you seek by consciously triggering the physical sensations of courage.

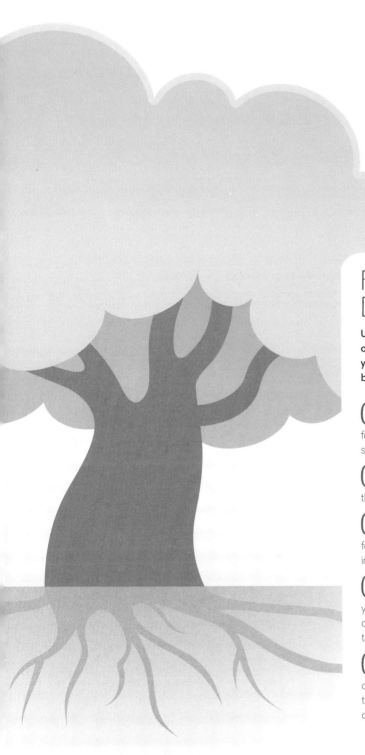

FOCUS ON DEVELOPING COURAGE

Use this technique whenever you notice an opportunity to practise the personal strength you wish to develop. Here we look at courage, but you can adapt it for any virtue.

01 When you notice an opportunity to practise courage, for example, when a situation creates fear or anxiety in you, recognize the bodily sensations of "no-courage".

02 Notice the mode of "no-courage": "I can't do this. Something bad will happen and then there will be trouble."

03 Use your willpower to develop the mode of courage physically by triggering the bodily feeling of courage: imagine a sense of expansion in your chest and energy in your muscles.

04 Consciously develop the mental and emotional mode of courage by telling yourself: "Taking this action might bring discomfort or loss, but it's the right thing to do and what I want to do." Hold onto these feelings, despite your fear.

05 Take action based on the mode of courage that you have just developed in your body and mind. Even if the fear is still there, you are able to proceed with courage, because that's where you are focusing your attention.

MEDITATION FOR THE
WORKPLACE AND PERFORMANCE

A toolset of practices

Whatever you do for a living, meditation gives you clarity, focus, and perspective, and improves your wellbeing – all of which are crucial if you want to succeed at work while finding balance and enjoying life.

One of the most common reasons people seek meditation is to improve their performance in their work. Many employers are also embracing meditation due to its proven abilities to increase productivity and decrease work-related stress.

By increasing your powers of attention and focus (see pp.22–23), and improving your mental clarity (see pp.148–149), meditating every day will gradually enhance your performance and wellbeing at work. But if you want to be more proactive and deliberate in this area, and accelerate the process, it can help to build the key skills of relaxation, awareness, and focus into your work day.

RELAXING AND DECOMPRESSING

● **Pre-meeting pause.** Have a 1-minute break before meetings, when you are sitting silently and just observing your body and breath.
● **Gaze away.** Take your eyes away from the task at hand and gaze at the horizon through your window to relax your mind and your eyes.
● **Take a breath.** In peaks of stress and anxiety during your work day, practise 5 minutes of alternate nostril breathing (see pp.168–169).

FOCUS ON DE-STRESSING

This Progressive Muscle Relaxation (PMR) technique helps you to relax when you feel tense and stressed during your day. You can practise it at your desk, or in a toilet break. If you have an injury, consult your doctor first.

01 If you can, sit down as this will help you relax more easily. Then, take a deep breath in while contracting all of the muscles in one leg and foot, and hold it for 5–10 seconds.

02 Breathe out while releasing all of the physical tension in your leg and foot. This will create a feeling of deep release, which can be hard to achieve by just trying to relax.

03 Pause briefly, taking one full breath, then repeat with the other leg and foot.

04 Repeat for the rest of your body, beginning at the bottom and working your way up: buttocks, stomach, each hand, arm, and shoulder, then your neck and face.

"Integrating meditation into your work day improves both your practice and performance."

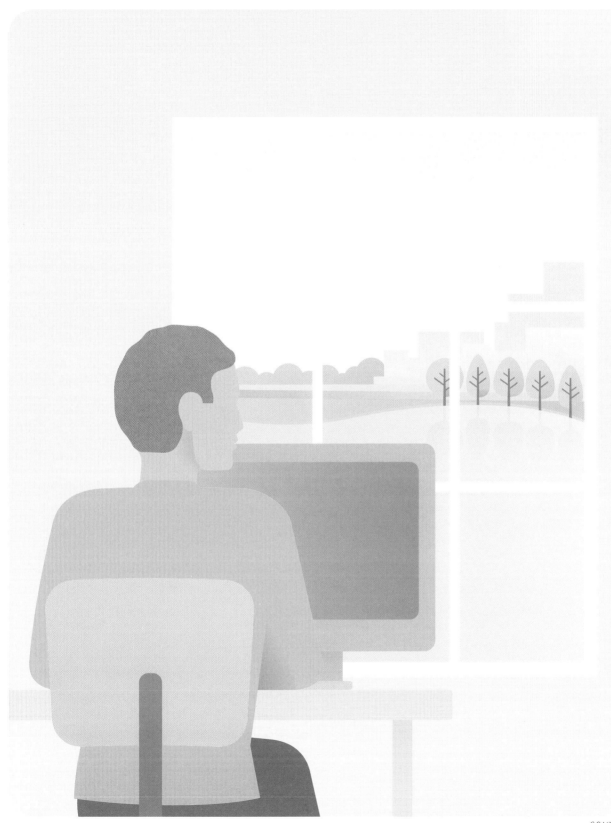

MEDITATION FOR THE WORKPLACE AND PERFORMANCE

CONTINUED ▶

154

EXPANDING AWARENESS

● **Lunch break.** Take 5–10 minutes in your lunch break, before eating, to sit down quietly and practise your favourite meditation, perhaps in a nearby park, or in an empty room in your workplace.

● **Informal walking meditation.** As you are walking to talk to someone, or to attend a meeting, or even to get some coffee, make it a mindful walk. Log out from the thinking mind for those few moments and simply pay attention to your feet touching the floor, or your breathing as you walk.

● **Mindful communication.** Talking to others is a good opportunity to practise self-awareness. When communicating with people, observe yourself by asking these four questions: What is the state of your mind as you speak and listen? Is your body tense and jumpy, or present and relaxed? How are your words, tone of voice, and facial expressions affecting your listener(s)? Are you really listening?

SHARPENING YOUR FOCUS

● **Work as meditation.** Treat the activity that you are engaged in at work as a meditation practice. This means that, when doing it, be 100 per cent present and focused, moment after moment. Continuously brush aside any distractions, just as you would let go of distracting thoughts during meditation.

● **Avoid multitasking.** Apply the above guidelines to one single task at a time. Multitasking cognitive tasks is not only ineffective from a productivity point of view, but it is also training your mind to be restless and unfocused.

● **Reduce distractions.** Adjust your environment so that it enables concentration, rather than distraction. For example, avoid having papers and objects out of place on your desk or in your workspace. Don't take your phone to meetings. If you work on a computer, only have open the documents, software, and browser tabs that you need to complete the work you are doing right now.

Reclaim your lunch break
Taking time away from your workspace during the day can make you more productive.

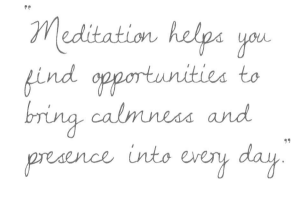

"Meditation helps you find opportunities to bring calmness and presence into every day."

WORKPLACE WELLBEING

FOR IMPROVING RELATIONSHIPS with your colleagues, try practising Loving-Kindness Meditation (see pp.134–135) and have them as the object.

TO PREPARE FOR TOUGH MEETINGS or challenges, use visualization before starting your work (see pp.146–147).

TO DEAL WITH STRONG EMOTIONS that arise, try managing them meditatively (see pp.144–145).

AFTER A LONG DAY SITTING AT A DESK, consider dynamic forms of meditation such as Yoga Asanas (see pp.94–95), Tai Chi (see pp.96–97), Kinhin (see pp.90–91), or the deeply relaxing Yoga Nidra (see pp.92–93).

MEDITATION FOR ATHLETES

Mastering the mental game

Whatever your sport, the path to success is filled with many mental obstacles – from losing motivation to having your energy hijacked by anxiety and worry. Meditation helps you master your mind, so you can master your game.

In a way, mastering your sport is about learning to fall in love with repetition: you need to be able to repeat the same drill again and again, each time with full focus and energy, without giving in to distracting thoughts or negative emotions, and without losing motivation. This is exactly what meditation does at a mental level.

Meditation also helps to increase your mental resilience to frustration, pain, stress, and tough training, improve sleep and reduce recovery times, and boost self-discipline – all of which enhance your athletic abilities.

A daily practice of any technique is likely to give you many of the benefits you seek, but if you want to improve specific areas, start with the list below:
● **Willpower and concentration:** Zazen (p.84), Trataka (p.102), Third Eye (p.108).
● **Motivation and self-confidence:** Vipassana (p.86), Mini-meditation 1 (p.44), Third Eye (p.108).
● **Relationship with teammates:** Mindfulness (p.82), Loving-Kindness (p.134), Labelling (p.112).

"With meditation, your sport can become a tool of personal growth and self-actualization."

FOCUS ON GETTING IN THE ZONE

01 Sit on a bench or chair, with your spine and neck straight and unsupported.

02 Spend a minute feeling your whole body, outside and inside. Feel its weight and shape. Your body is your highly trained tool: let your mind become one with it, become intimate with it. Ask for its full commitment for the important moments that will come up. Feel it becoming extremely strong, flexible, and quick.

03 Move your attention to your breath. Breathe in deeply through your nose, counting to 5, then hold your breath for 10 seconds. Breathe out, counting to 5. If you find this too easy and it doesn't require enough focus, try inhaling for 7 seconds, holding for 14, then exhaling for 7.

04 Relax inside your breathing: with each inhalation, feel that you are filling yourself with energy, power, and strength. While holding your breath, feel that power permeate every muscle of your body. When exhaling, release all fear, all worry, all tiredness.

05 Follow this breathing for 4–5 minutes. End the meditation here, and go forward confidently. Or, if you have time, spend 5–10 minutes visualizing yourself succeeding in your goal (see pp.146–147).

157

MEDITATION FOR ATHLETES

MEDITATION FOR PUBLIC SPEAKERS

Calming the nerves

Whether it's a presentation at work, an interview, or a wedding speech, most of us will need to speak in front of an audience at some point in our lives. This can be extremely daunting, but meditation can help stop our nerves getting the best of us.

For many people, the most challenging thing about public speaking is to control their nerves. When dominated by fear, anxiety, or nervousness, our voice can be shaky or weak, or we speak too quickly, which limits our impact. We might also move around nervously, distracting the audience, or we are meek and have no stage presence. We may even panic and forget our speech altogether.

Calmness is essential for a good speech, so when you're building up to a speech or presentation, choose meditations that emphasize relaxation or awareness, and that work with your breathing and body. If your nerves come from a fear of forgetting your speech, practise meditation techniques that emphasize concentration. You can also use visualization as a tool to overcome feelings of nervousness (see pp.146–147).

During your speech, be aware of whatever thoughts and emotions arise, but use the breathing and awareness skills you have developed to anchor yourself in your body, in the present moment. Nervousness and anxiety may still arise, but you will still feel in control, and deliver an excellent speech.

FOCUS ON CALMING THE NERVES

If you feel anxious before giving a speech, this breathing technique, known as box breathing, will help you feel calm, confident, and ready to perform. You can do it without anyone even noticing.

01 Keep your eyes open or closed – whichever feels most comfortable. Whether you are standing or sitting, keep your neck and back upright and straight.

02 Breathe in through your nose counting for 4 seconds. Hold your breath for 4 seconds.

03 Breathe out through your nose for 4 seconds, then wait for another 4 seconds before breathing in for 4 seconds again.

04 Let each breath be slow, deep, and even, and make sure your breathing is abdominal.

05 Repeat this for 10–20 cycles. If you find 4 seconds too difficult, try starting with 3 seconds and increasing after a couple of rounds. If it's too easy and doesn't take up enough of your focus, use 5 or 6 seconds.

"With daily meditation, you can keep calm and confident when delivering your speech."

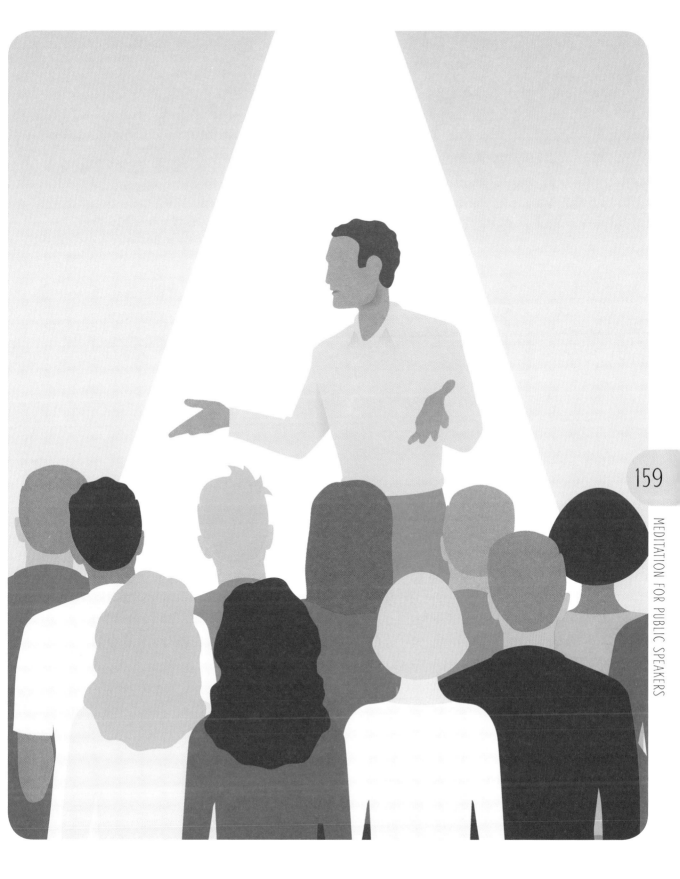

MEDITATION FOR CREATIVITY

Inspiration from beyond

Creativity is a wonderful human ability, but it can easily become suffocated by a busy mind or patterns of thinking that are overly rational or literal. Meditation helps declutter your thoughts and inspire you, no matter how you want to use creativity in your life.

Have you ever struggled to be creative, or to find a solution to a problem, only to think of the answer once you had forgotten all about it? We often need this "letting go" for our creativity to flourish, which is exactly where meditation can help.

To develop this state, practise techniques that emphasize awareness, or open monitoring practices, such as Mindfulness (see pp.82–83) or Vipassana (see pp.86–87). By inviting us to pay non-judgmental attention to whatever arises and develop awareness of everything around us, open monitoring practices promote divergent thinking, improve our ability to notice new things, and foster openness to experience in general, all of which are essential to creativity.

Choose visualization meditations if you want to be visually creative, or sound-based practices if you are a musician or composer. For general creative thinking, select practices that stimulate intuition, such as Third Eye (see pp.108–109) and Zazen (see pp.84–85), or deep relaxation.

"*Meditation helps create the optimal mental state for creativity to flourish.*"

FOCUS ON GETTING YOUR JUICES FLOWING

Try this meditation to get in the zone creatively. Before you start, contemplate an inspiring piece of work from an artist in your field, such as a painting, song, or poem.

01 Sit in a comfortable posture and close your eyes. Take three deep breaths through your nose. With every out-breath, allow your body to become more relaxed and still. Close your mouth and relax into the present moment.

02 Try to reproduce the piece of work you have chosen in your mind: make it as vivid as you can. Let that masterpiece permeate your whole awareness. Let your mind become one with it. Study its beauty and uncover its mysteries. Try to imagine and feel the state of mind the creator was in while they created it.

03 Bring your focus back to yourself and remember a moment in your life when inspiration was flowing. How were you feeling at that moment? What state were your body, mind, and heart in? Try to relive that experience.

04 Bring your next creative challenge to mind. Contemplate it like an empty canvas waiting to be filled. Channel the inspiration you've fostered and let that flow into this empty canvas.

05 When you feel it flowing, open your eyes, and make your art a reality.

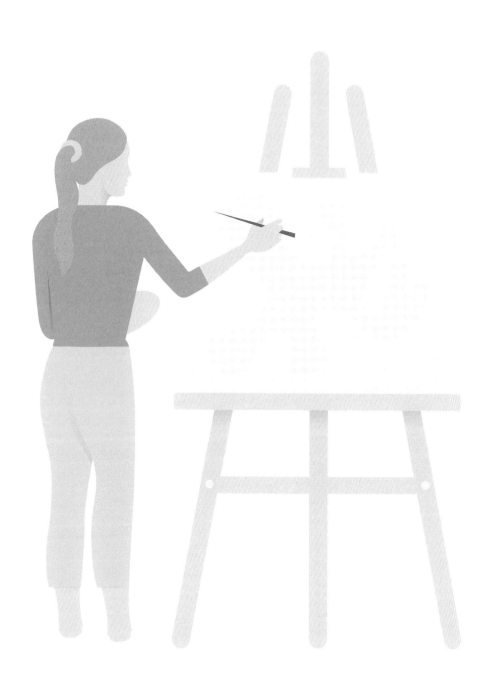

A NEW LEVEL

Going deeper in your practice

Meditation is a continual journey – there is always more to learn or experience about yourself and your practice. Once you've established meditation as a strong daily habit, you might be asking yourself: "What next?"

After practising the same meditation technique every day for several months, many meditators begin to feel as though they aren't making as much progress anymore. This is completely normal. You can try any of the following ideas to help you go deeper in your practice. Choose whichever are most practical for you.

MEDITATE FOR LONGER

There are no fixed rules for how long your sessions should be, but a general guideline is to arrive at a point where you meditate for at least 20 minutes per session, every day. If you already do that, you can try increasing this to 30–40 minutes. However, if you are seeking the spiritual benefits of meditation (see pp.28–29 and pp.176–177), many teachers recommend that your daily session lasts for at least 40 minutes to one hour.

FOCUS ON QUALITY OVER QUANTITY

You can improve the quality of your meditation in two ways: by increasing its intensity, and by preparing for your practice.

To increase the intensity of your practice, have a strong intention to really give yourself fully to your practice. We pay attention to what we consider important, so make sure you are taking it seriously. Mastering the art of concentration will also help you to generate some of that inner fire (see pp.74–75).

Just as you need to warm up before exercising, calming your body and centring your mind will help you achieve the optimal state for meditation:

● **Alternate nostril breathing** (see pp.168–169), Humming Bee Pranayama (pp.88–89), and Mini-meditation 1 (pp.44–45) calm your body and breath.
● **Incorporating an element** of ritual into your practice helps to centre your mind (see pp.164–165).

INTEGRATE MEDITATION INTO YOUR DAY

The quality of your meditation influences your daily life, but the quality of your mind in daily life also influences your meditation. Keep your mind less busy and restless during the day by integrating pauses and mini-meditations into your life, and making your activities meditative (see pp.140–141).

CONNECT MORE DEEPLY WITH THE PRACTICE

Spend time reflecting on your practice and learning more about it so it becomes a greater part of your life. You can try:

- **Journalling** your experiences and progress.
- **Reading** around the subject (see pp.182–184).
- **Joining a meditation group** and spending time with other meditators.
- **Finding a meditation teacher** that you can talk to, be inspired by, and ask questions.
- **Going to** a meditation retreat (see pp.174–175).

"Going deeper in your practice will enable you to get the most out of it."

RESPECTING THE SESSION

Introducing an element of ritual

Creating a ritual around an activity or event helps to mark it as important. By surrounding it with an atmosphere of reverence, you ensure that you pay attention to it – which is exactly what mindfulness is about.

We often think of rituals as something religious, but secular culture has many rituals too, such as birthdays or graduation ceremonies. Introducing a form of ritual to your meditation practice, however simple, sends a message to yourself that it is something important. This helps you focus your mind and heart in the practice more deeply.

Zen practitioners, for example, bow to their meditation cushion before starting a session. This is to remind themselves: "I'm about to do something important, something worthy of respect. Be present! Sitting here is different from sitting on my sofa in front of the television!"

GOING DEEPER

Rituals are not essential to meditation, but they can help you have a deeper meditation experience, so are something that you can consider adopting once your meditation habit is already well established. By surrounding your practice with something that is meaningful to you, you also bring more calm and pause to the rest of your day.

Your meditation rituals can be as simple or as elaborate, as secular or as spiritual as you like (see opposite). They can be deeply personal, and you may want to keep them private.

"Rituals are tools to channel your thoughts and emotions into creating a specific result in yourself or the world."

EVERYDAY RITUALS

Try using any of the following ideas to create a sense of importance around your meditation practice, and to bring more pause and calm into your day.

Before your meditation, you can try:
WASHING your hands and face.
PUTTING ON a specific set of clothes that are comfortable for the practice.
LIGHTING some incense or a candle.
SETTING your intentions for the practice.

A post-meditation ritual could be:
WRITING in a journal.
DRINKING a cup of tea while taking time to reflect.
GOING for a calm and mindful walk.
PRACTISING some affirmations.
SETTING your intentions for the day.

OVERCOMING THE HINDRANCES TO MEDITATION

Finding room for improvement

If you feel you aren't getting the maximum benefit from your practice, try looking over the hindrances shown here to identify where to focus your effort for improvement: sometimes just recognizing a hindrance will diminish its power over you.

Traditional philosophies, particularly from the Buddhist and Yogic traditions, identify different mental states that can stop you going deep in your meditation. Recognizing these hindrances and learning how to overcome them is an important part of growing your practice.

These mental states are a completely normal part of the journey and they are likely to be the companions of your meditation for a long time. Simply develop your awareness of them and follow the suggested solutions to the best of your ability: for most, it is enough to continue the practice with patience, perseverance, and energy, but others have more specific solutions. Any progress you make is worth celebrating!

Deepen your understanding of your practice and consult a teacher (see pp.182–184).

Try introducing an element of ritual to create a greater sense of importance around it (see pp.164–165).

> " Tackling these obstacles is all about awareness and taking baby steps."

Progressing on the path
The obstacles and solutions shown here are inspired by those identified in the Yogic and Buddhist traditions.

166

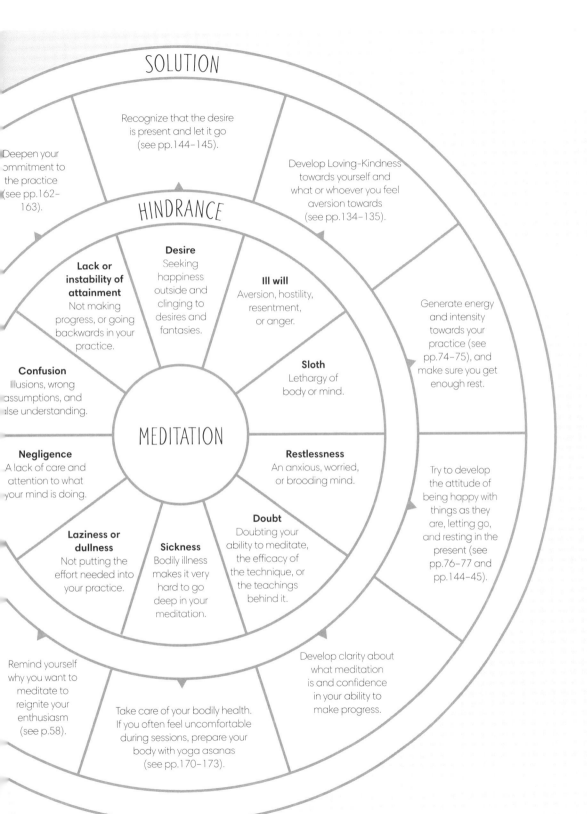

SOLUTION

HINDRANCE

MEDITATION

Recognize that the desire is present and let it go (see pp.144–145).

Deepen your commitment to the practice (see pp.162–163).

Develop Loving-Kindness towards yourself and what or whoever you feel aversion towards (see pp.134–135).

Generate energy and intensity towards your practice (see pp.74–75), and make sure you get enough rest.

Try to develop the attitude of being happy with things as they are, letting go, and resting in the present (see pp.76–77 and pp.144–45).

Develop clarity about what meditation is and confidence in your ability to make progress.

Take care of your bodily health. If you often feel uncomfortable during sessions, prepare your body with yoga asanas (see pp.170–173).

Remind yourself why you want to meditate to reignite your enthusiasm (see p.58).

Lack or instability of attainment
Not making progress, or going backwards in your practice.

Desire
Seeking happiness outside and clinging to desires and fantasies.

Ill will
Aversion, hostility, resentment, or anger.

Sloth
Lethargy of body or mind.

Restlessness
An anxious, worried, or brooding mind.

Doubt
Doubting your ability to meditate, the efficacy of the technique, or the teachings behind it.

Sickness
Bodily illness makes it very hard to go deep in your meditation.

Laziness or dullness
Not putting the effort needed into your practice.

Negligence
A lack of care and attention to what your mind is doing.

Confusion
Illusions, wrong assumptions, and false understanding.

167

OVERCOMING THE HINDRANCES TO MEDITATION

SUPERCHARGE YOUR PRACTICE

Alternate nostril breathing

Practising some simple breathing exercises before meditation will help deepen your session. Alternate nostril breathing (*nadi shodhana*), shown here, is one of the most popular and effective techniques from the Yogic tradition.

In alternate nostril breathing you use the thumb and index finger of your right hand to close and open your nostrils so you only breathe through one nostril at a time. Following this technique, shown right, for 3–4 minutes will calm your body, stabilize your nervous system, and make your mind clearer. This makes alternate nostril breathing an excellent preparation for meditation and an effective way to create moments of calm in your day, or to manage overwhelming emotions.

BREATHING GUIDELINES

During the practice, make sure that your breathing is abdominal (see pp.70–71) and through your nose. Your breath should be:

● **Slow.** Take your time – there is no need to hurry.
● **Deep.** When inhaling, take in plenty of air. When exhaling, empty your lungs completely.
● **Steady.** The quantity of air you inhale should be constant throughout the inhalation, as if you were smoothly filling a bottle with water. The same goes for the exhalation.

At no time should you feel the need to pause and take a few normal breaths. If you do, start the exercise again with a breath length that you are more comfortable with, keeping the exhalation double the length of the inhalation. The longer your breaths, the stronger the effect of this practice, but keep it natural – you should finish feeling calm and energized, not panting for air!

01 Sit down comfortably wherever you are. If you are doing this as a preparation before your main practice, you can sit in the meditation posture.

02 You can keep your eyes open, but it is better to close them for a deeper relaxation.

03 Breathe in deeply through your nose, then release your breath fully in a long exhalation, producing a slight "haaa" sound through your mouth. Then close your mouth.

04 Bend your index and middle fingers so they reach the base of your thumb. Close your right nostril using your right thumb, and inhale through your left nostril, counting 1, 2, 3.

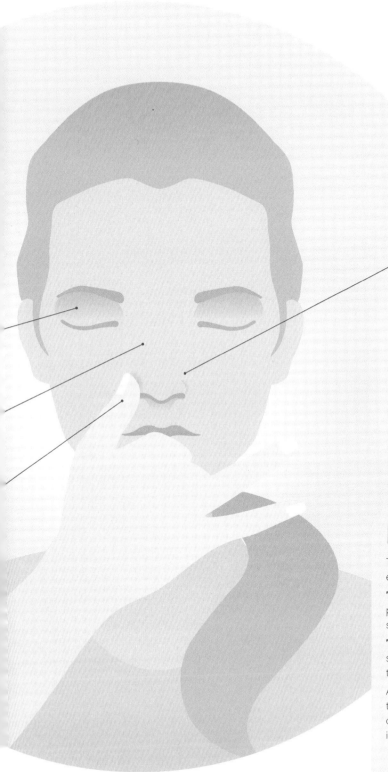

05 Close your left nostril with the ring finger on your right hand and open your right nostril. Exhale counting 1, 2, 3, 4, 5, 6.

06 Breathe in through your right nostril counting to 3, then close your right nostril, open the left nostril, and breathe out counting to 6. This completes one round of the breathing. Practise 10–20 rounds.

07 If breathing in for 3 seconds and out for 6 is hard, you can try 2 in and 4 out. If it is easy, increase the length, always keeping the exhalation twice the length of the inhalation.

08 Notice the difference in your body and mind. Relax your raised arm, close your eyes if they aren't already, and proceed with your meditation. Or, open your eyes and conclude the practice.

BREATHING FOR BALANCE

The Yogic tradition includes many breathing exercises called pranayama. They teach that:

THE LEFT NOSTRIL is connected to the parasympathetic nervous system, and right side of the brain.

THE RIGHT NOSTRIL is connected to the sympathetic nervous system, and left side of the brain.

As a result, by alternating your breath between the nostrils, you achieve a greater balance and relaxation of the nervous system and more interaction between the two brain hemispheres.

PREPARING FOR LONGER SESSIONS

Yoga asanas for meditation

With the right posture and props, you should be able to sit comfortably in meditation for 20 minutes. But if you want to meditate for longer, or start going to retreats, you will need to prepare your body.

Yoga asanas, or postures, were originally developed to keep the body healthy, flexible, and strong in preparation for deep meditation. They help you to:

● **Develop flexibility** in the hips and knees. The more flexible your hips and knees are, the more stable and relaxed you will feel in meditation.

● **Strengthen the back muscles,** enabling you to keep your back and neck straight for longer as they are the only muscles that you don't relax fully during seated meditation.

● **Release tensions** and allow you to relax more deeply, helping to release mental tensions too.

Practise the asanas shown here, following the guidelines on the right, to prepare your body for longer sessions. You can also try other asanas under the guidance of a Yoga teacher, and may want to include a spinal twist. If you have health concerns, consult your doctor first.

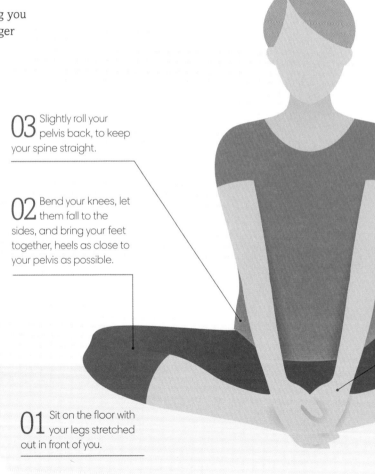

03 Slightly roll your pelvis back, to keep your spine straight.

02 Bend your knees, let them fall to the sides, and bring your feet together, heels as close to your pelvis as possible.

FULL BUTTERFLY OR BOUND ANGLE POSE
(Poorna titali asana or Baddha konasana) This asana improves hip and groin flexibility. If your hips or lower back are stiff, sit on a folded blanket.

01 Sit on the floor with your legs stretched out in front of you.

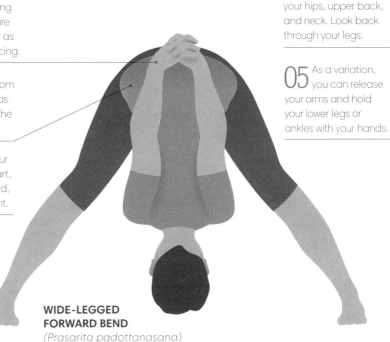

03 When you have reached your limit, straighten your arms behind your back, clasp your hands together, and bring them forward so your arms are perpendicular to the floor, or as close as possible without forcing.

02 Slowly bend forward from the hips, going as far as comfortable, while keeping the back elongated.

01 Stand with your legs wide apart, toes pointing forward, and back up straight.

04 Hold the final position and breathe deeply. Relax your hips, upper back, and neck. Look back through your legs.

05 As a variation, you can release your arms and hold your lower legs or ankles with your hands.

05 After a while, you can deepen the stretch by holding your feet and pressing your thighs towards the floor with your elbows. When you feel a good stretch, hold for a few seconds and breathe deeply.

04 Hold your feet with your hands and gently move your knees up and down 30–50 times, without pushing. Or, place your hands on your knees and use them to move your legs up and down.

WIDE-LEGGED FORWARD BEND
(Prasarita padottanasana)
This asana stretches, loosens, and relaxes the muscles along the spine. An alternative is Child's pose (see p.95).

HOW TO PRACTISE ASANAS

Perform these asanas according to your time and needs, bearing the following guidelines in mind. The poses should stretch you, but not cause you pain: be slow and mindful, and don't push your limits. If in doubt, consult your doctor and a Yoga teacher.

HOLD EACH POSE for at least 30 seconds.

IF YOU PRACTISE ASANAS that bend your back in one direction, follow with a posture that bends it in the opposite direction, for a similar amount of time.

ALWAYS END THE SESSION with a relaxation pose.

CONTINUED ▶

01 Sit with your legs stretched out in front of you and keep your feet together.

02 Slightly lift your body for a moment by pushing away from the ground with your hands, and roll your pelvis back to straighten the spine.

05 When you are ready, use your arms to help you come back up slowly.

172

SEATED FORWARD BEND
(Paschimottanasana)
This pose strengthens your back muscles. If this causes discomfort in your lower back, sit on a folded blanket.

03 Exhale and bend forward from the hips. Extend your arms forward and reach as far down the legs as you comfortably can.

04 Hold the position, breathing deeply and releasing tension in your hip, thigh, and back muscles with each out-breath.

01 Lie on your front, resting your forehead on the floor.

02 Stretch your arms forward, with your palms facing down.

03 Keep your legs straight and parallel, with your big toes touching each other.

04 Close your eyes, relax your whole body, and pay attention to your breathing, or your body as a whole.

REVERSED CORPSE POSE
(Advasana)
Use this deeply relaxing pose to finish your practice. An alternative is to lie on your back (see pp.68-69).

SHOULDER POSE

(Kandharasana)
Use this pose to strengthen the muscles in your lower back.

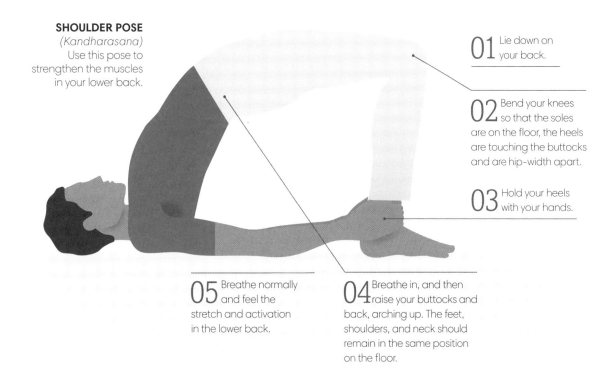

01 Lie down on your back.

02 Bend your knees so that the soles are on the floor, the heels are touching the buttocks and are hip-width apart.

03 Hold your heels with your hands.

05 Breathe normally and feel the stretch and activation in the lower back.

04 Breathe in, and then raise your buttocks and back, arching up. The feet, shoulders, and neck should remain in the same position on the floor.

SPHINX OR EASY COBRA POSE

(Saral bhujangasana)
This pose strengthens your upper back. An alternative is Crocodile pose (see p.95).

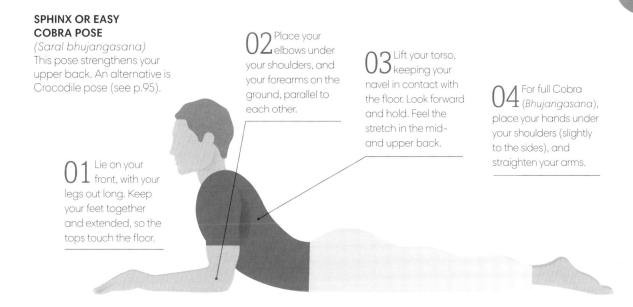

02 Place your elbows under your shoulders, and your forearms on the ground, parallel to each other.

03 Lift your torso, keeping your navel in contact with the floor. Look forward and hold. Feel the stretch in the mid- and upper back.

04 For full Cobra *(Bhujangasana)*, place your hands under your shoulders (slightly to the sides), and straighten your arms.

01 Lie on your front, with your legs out long. Keep your feet together and extended, so the tops touch the floor.

TO ADVANCE, RETREAT!

What to expect

A meditation retreat is one of the best ways to take your practice to the next level. Knowing what to expect and when to go will help you get the best out of the experience.

Retreats give you a pause in your life, allowing you to delve deep into meditation, free from the usual distractions, but they are not meant to be relaxing. They can bring up intense emotions, so make sure you are prepared for this and consider when is the right time for you to go. You are also likely to see part of yourself that you didn't know existed, and in a retreat there is no way to close your eyes to that. That is why retreats are good ground for deep introspection and transformation.

By gaining a deeper understanding of yourself, retreats help you cope better with the challenges of daily life. You may also become more aware of how your environment and other people affect your energy and mental states. This enhanced awareness empowers you to make concrete positive changes, such as distancing yourself from negative or unhelpful situations.

WHAT TO EXPECT

Everything in a retreat is designed so that you can focus exclusively on your meditation. Each has different practices, rules, and approaches, so research your options thoroughly. However, many retreats do share the following elements:

● **Duration.** For a smoother experience, a retreat of 1–3 days is best for beginners, though some can last 5–10 days or more. Whatever its length, you are usually asked to stay for the full duration.

● **Routine.** A set routine promotes a simple lifestyle, in which it is always clear what you are supposed to do next. This enables your mind to be empty and present, which supports your meditation. To stop the mind wandering, retreats fill each day with meditation and related activities, such as Yoga.

● **Food.** To support your physical wellbeing, retreats often only provide healthy vegetarian food and snacks at set times. This is designed to help you feel lighter in your body and save energy that would otherwise be used in additional digestion.

● **Lodging.** Though private rooms are occasionally available, retreats give you an opportunity to jump out of your comfort zone and try a simple and communal lifestyle by providing shared rooms, often with two or four people of the same gender.

● **Silence.** Your deepening in meditation is greatly facilitated by the rule of silence, which is usually followed for part of the day or the entire retreat. Everything is organized so that you don't need to speak to anyone.

● **Reading.** To enable you to fully face yourself and digest your experiences, many retreats discourage reading, as this feeds the mind with new concepts and ideas.

● **Devices.** To maintain the focus, presence, and clarity that are built up through meditation, the use of computers, mobile phones, and tablets is not allowed.

● **Cleaning.** Many retreats encourage you to practise meditation in daily life activities through group cleaning. In Zen this is called *samu* and in Yoga it is *karma yoga*.

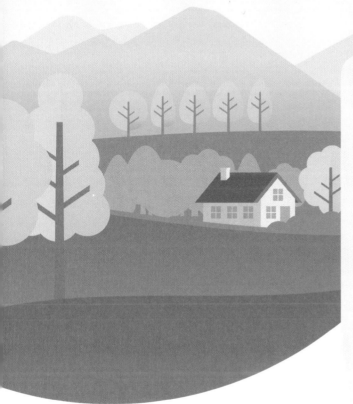

"Retreats give you deep self-understanding and sharper tools to work with your mind and emotions."

WHAT TO LOOK FOR

If you're new to meditation, a retreat can be overwhelming. But if you have established a daily practice over several months, and wish to take it further, it can be a very beneficial experience. Whatever stage you're at, consider these guidelines:

START SMALL. Try shorter 1 to 3-day retreats before going to longer ones.

SEEK CONNECTION. Some retreats are secular, but most are run by spiritual groups. Choose a retreat that includes the practice you follow and is led by a teacher or group that you respect and can connect with.

BE OPEN. When participating in a retreat, keep your mind open, non-judgmental, and willing. Dropping all expectations, and having patience and flexibility, will help you get the most out of your experience.

MORE TO LIFE

Meditation as a spiritual path

Over the last century, meditation has become largely separated from its religious roots. But as you recognize its positive impact on your body and mind, you might wonder if its spiritual origins could have something equally valuable to offer.

For some people, meditation is about more than its health and wellbeing benefits – it is part of a spiritual lifestyle and a whole new way of seeing the world. If that is something you'd like to explore, the advice on these pages will help you get started.

EMBRACING THE SPIRITUAL SIDE

Put simply, spirituality is the belief that there is more to life than what meets the senses, more to the universe than purposeless mechanics, more to consciousness than electrical impulses in the brain, and more to our existence than the body and its physical needs.

From that point of view, meditation practice can have the aim of spiritual growth, development, purification, or liberation – though this can depend on which tradition you adopt (see pp.20–21).

CHOOSING YOUR PATH

Just as you are guided to discover the meditation technique that best matches your personality and goals, you can explore different aspects of spirituality by experiencing different ideas, books, teachers, and groups, and seeing where you feel most at home. A good way to start can be to explore the traditions behind the practices you enjoy.

As you embark on your spiritual journey, it's worth bearing in mind the following guidelines:

● **Different traditions** may have contrasting theories and practices. Experience several different paths so that you can compare them. Remember that no single approach is best for everyone.

● **It may be helpful** to try different teachers or approaches, even within the same tradition.

● **See how you feel** in each group, and listen to your gut and heart.

● **Observe the teacher** and more experienced students: do they embody the qualities and knowledge that you are looking for?

● **As you progress,** you may find that what was once helpful no longer is. Know that you are able to change your path if you want to.

"Pursuing the spiritual side of meditation can give a new sense of meaning to your life."

IS IT FOR ME?

Read over the following goals of meditation as a spiritual practice – if any of them speak deeply to you, it's likely that you would benefit from exploring the spiritual side of your practice.

PURIFYING THE MIND AND HEART of illusions and negative patterns.

DISCOVERING AND ACTUALIZING your true Self (Consciousness or Spirit).

SURRENDERING AND UNITING with the Divine, in whichever form you take this to be.

UPROOTING ALL DELUSION and seeing reality as it is.

ACHIEVING SPIRITUAL ENLIGHTENMENT, liberation, or awakening.

DISSOLVING THE EGO OR PERSONALITY, like a drop merging with the ocean.

HARMONIZING YOURSELF with the Spirit or Tao.

FREEING YOURSELF from the earthly cycle of birth and death.

To learn more about the spiritual benefits of meditation, see Practical Spirituality (pp.28-29).

CONNECTING WITH THE DIVINE

Meditation and devotion

One of meditation's many spiritual purposes is devotion. If you're interested in this side of your practice, devotional meditation, such as Kirtan, can be a powerful means of spiritual connection.

While some traditions see the spiritual purpose of meditation as purifying oneself or liberating the mind from suffering, others, including Christian Mysticism and the Hindu Bhakti Yoga, see meditation as a means of devotion. This means to focus the heart and mind on the Divine while developing strong religious feeling and surrender, making it a powerful way to explore the spiritual side of your practice.

In Christian Mysticism, for example, meditation helps keep the mind and heart focused on God by repeating a sacred word or sentence, or by focusing on a feeling of Divine presence. The Hindu approach includes similar practices, as well as a practice of group chanting called Kirtan, which is gaining popularity in a more secularized form in the West. The Sikh tradition also includes a practice of Kirtan chanting. Kirtan is a particularly good introduction to devotional meditation as it gives you a direct taste of emotional surrender, without asking you to believe in anything specific.

DEVOTIONAL SINGING

Kirtan is a call-and-response chant of the "names of the Divine", usually sung in Sanskrit or Hindi. It uses the flow of music and emotions to bypass the mind, and arrive at a state of stillness or even ecstasy.

As one of the main practices of Bhakti Yoga, the Yoga of the heart, Kirtan aims to awaken the feeling of *bhakti* in the heart, leading to an altered state of consciousness. *Bhakti* is a feeling of devotion and surrender to a higher spiritual ideal, whatever name and shape you want to give it. The more *bhakti* is developed in you, the more uplifted you feel, giving you a sense of ease, wonder, and bliss. Kirtan also enhances your sensitivity and soothes the mind. To start with, the best way to experience Kirtan is by joining a session at a yoga or meditation studio. It is helpful to keep the following guidelines in mind:

● **Attitude.** *Bhava* – the emotion and attitude behind singing – is the most important element of Kirtan. It brings about the opening of the heart, and the release and channelling of your emotions.

"Kirtan helps you connect to something deeper inside yourself. You are singing for the awakening of your own heart."

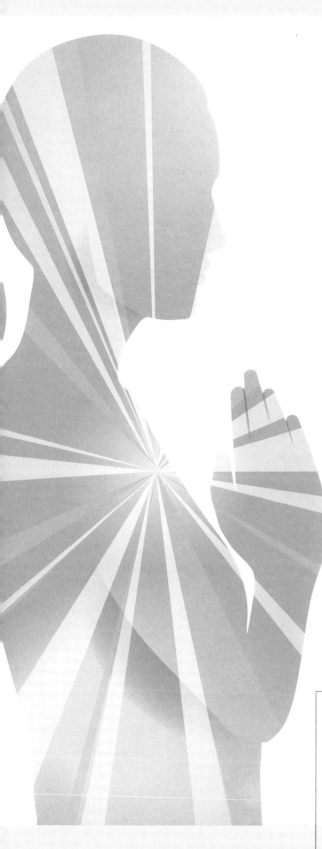

- **Openness.** Kirtan leads you to leave the realm of the mind and to connect from a place of openness and surrender, so you might feel a bit uncomfortable at first. This makes it important to choose a group setting in which you feel safe.
- **Non-judgment.** Your mind may be telling you that your voice is bad, or group singing is odd, but you will only have a real experience of what Kirtan can do for you by suspending all judgment for the duration of the session.
- **Heartfulness.** Sound and voice are the vehicles of emotion; the mind just gets in the way. Leave your intellect at the door and allow yourself to experience whatever feelings may come up. Open your heart, be there completely, and let Kirtan lead the way into what might be a new and mysterious place for you.

After a few songs, you may arrive at a space full of silence, openness, and heartfulness. If that happens, you can continue to sit or stand in silence, and enjoy the meditation.

Getting connected
If you are seeking spiritual connection from meditation, you may want to experiment with devotional techniques.

SAMADHI

The zenith of complete mental mastery

How far can meditation take you? What kind of mental states and experiences can be achieved through it? Several contemplative traditions describe the ultimate state of meditation as *samadhi,* a state of perfect mental mastery.

There are varying definitions of *samadhi,* but in the Yogic and Vedic traditions, *samadhi* is a state of absorption equivalent to what the Buddhists call *jhanna.* There are several different levels of *samadhi,* but according to their classical definition, they all have the following in common:

● **Complete and uninterrupted union** of consciousness with the meditation object. Mind and object become one, without any duality. Eventually, when even that object disappears or becomes more subtle, a deeper level of *samadhi* opens up effortlessly.

● **Complete and continuous thoughtlessness** and stillness of mind. Not a single thought, memory, or image appears in the mind for several minutes, or even hours.

● **No awareness of the environment,** as if the senses have temporarily been shut down. Someone could call your name, and you wouldn't even hear it.

● **No awareness of your body.** Your consciousness has temporarily freed itself from the limitations of, and identification with, your body, and yet is fully aware. Your body could be in pain, but you wouldn't notice.

In *samadhi* the individuality or ego is not functioning. In this state, you undergo deep purification of the conscious and unconscious mind, returning transformed and unable to explain what has just happened to you.

In both Buddhism and Yoga, *samadhi* is the culmination of concentration practices, but it is not the same as enlightenment. Instead, it is the highest tool, or practice, to achieve that ultimate goal.

Although you will experience the benefits of meditation without reaching or even nearing *samadhi,* it is important to know about it. Achieving *samadhi* is an incredibly ambitious aim, and some meditation teachers have now either de-emphasized it, or talk about it in much more achievable terms. It's best to think of it as direction and inspiration for your practice.

THE JOURNEY OF SAMADHI

With each level of *samadhi*, the objects and mental states become increasingly subtle. In the Yogic tradition, for example, there are eight levels of *samadhi* "with an object" (*sabija samadhi*), starting with "gross" or physical objects, such as the breath or a candle flame, and going as subtle as consciousness itself (the essence of "I am"). After this, there is the "objectless absorption" (*nirbija samadhi*). Likewise, Buddhism talks about the *jhannas* of form and the formless *jhannas*.

This final state of samadhi is very rare, even among monks and other very experienced meditators. Having a glimpse of it is one thing, while the ability to enter it at will is something else entirely.

"Samadhi is a state of unshakable peace, direct knowledge, and supreme bliss."

RESOURCES

GENERAL INFORMATION

Meditation and its Practice (Swami Rama)
A short and accessible introduction to the several aspects of meditation practice, by a well-known Yogi.

How to Meditate: A Practical Guide to Making Friends with Your Mind (Pema Chödrön)
Learn how to explore and work with the mind and emotions.

Meditation for Beginners (Jack Kornfield)
An easy-to-follow introduction to eight different types of Buddhist meditation.

LiveAndDare
The author's blog, covering a series of meditation-related topics in-depth in a pragmatic and non-sectarian way.
liveanddare.com

Wildmind
A secular presentation of different types of Buddhist meditation.
wildmind.org

Mindful
A friendly, secular blog covering many aspects of Mindfulness Meditation, including a digital magazine.
mindful.org

YOGIC MEDITATION & PHILOSOPHY

Sure Ways to Self-Realization (Swami Satyananda Saraswati)
An in-depth work about the different types of meditation from the Yoga tradition, as well as many others, including Inner Silence (*Antar Mouna*), Mantra (*Japa*), Yoga Nidra, Trataka, and Kundalini (*Kriya Yoga*). A "must-read" for any meditator that enjoys Yogic techniques.

Asana Pranayama Mudra Bandha (Swami Satyananda Saraswati)
An extensive collection of Yoga asanas (postures) and pranayama (breathing exercises), explained in an accessible way alongside the background theory.

Path of Fire and Light: Volume 2 (Swami Rama)
A short book covering Mantra, Kundalini, and breathing meditations, with a discussion about working with the mind and its patterns.

Mantra Yoga and Primal Sound: Secrets of Seed (Bija) Mantras (Dr David Frawley)
A thorough exploration of all aspects of Mantra practice.

Ajna Chakra (Rishi Nityabodhananda)
A short book about Third Eye Meditations and awakening.

Autobiography of a Yogi (Paramahansa Yogananda)
One of the most popular modern books of the Yoga tradition.

Vijnanabhairava or Divine Consciousness: A Treasury of 112 Types of Yoga (Jaideva Singh)
A modern translation and commentary on a Tantric text that describes over a hundred different types of meditation.

The Yoga Tradition: Its History, Literature, Philosophy and Practice (Georg Feuerstein)
A treatise on the history, philosophy, and practice of several Yoga lineages.

The Living Gita: The Complete Bhagavad Gita (Swami Satchidananda)
A modern translation of one of the cornerstone spiritual texts of India.

Yoga Forums
The largest online forum for all things solely Yoga-related, including Yogic meditation techniques and pranayama (breathing exercises).
yogaforums.com

Bihar Yoga
This website, from the gurus of Bihar Yoga, makes ancient secret practices of Yoga openly available and simple to follow.
biharyoga.net

Traditional Yoga Studies
For those who want a deeper understanding of the history and philosophy of Yoga.
traditionalyogastudies.com

Himalayan Institute
A legacy of Swami Rama, an important Yogi who travelled to the West in the 20th century.
himalayaninstitute.org

SwamiJ
A library of articles exploring the contemplative side of the Yoga and Tantric traditions.
swamij.com

VEDANTIC MEDITATION & PHILOSOPHY

Vedantic Meditation: Lighting the Flame of Awareness (David Frawley)
Accessible reading into the principles and practices of this tradition.

Advaita Made Easy (Dennis Waite)
Introduction to the topic of Vedic thought and non-duality.

I Am That (Nisargadatta Maharaj)
A modern spiritual classic that eloquently teaches the "I am" meditation technique.

Be As You Are: The Teachings of Sri Ramana Maharshi (ed. David Godman)
The best collection of teachings of the famous self-enquiry sage, Sri Ramana Maharshi.

The Heart of Awareness: A Translation of the Ashtavakra Gita (trans. Thomas Byrom)
Translation and commentary from the Ashtavakra Gita, expounding the philosophy of Advaita Vedanta.

Advaita Bodha Deepika (Sri Karapatra Swami)
A short classical text outlining the whole spiritual path of non-duality and self-enquiry.

Sri Ramana Maharshi
Ramana Maharshi was the first Indian guru to popularize the practice of Self-Enquiry meditation. This is his official website.
sriramanamaharshi.org

Nisargadatta Maharaj
Nisargadatta Maharaj is the author of the modern spiritual classic *I Am That*, and a master of the Self-Enquiry meditation technique.
nisargadatta.net

Avadhuta Foundation
The official website of H.W.L. Poonja, also known as Papaji, a famous guru who expounded the effortless path to awakening, with a Vedantic background.
avadhuta.com

Awakening Beyond Thought
The website of Gary Weber, a well-known Western teacher who exposes the path of Self-Enquiry in a clean and simple way.
happiness-beyond-thought.com

Vedanta Spiritual Library
A large online library of traditional texts about the Vedantic teachings and philosophy.
celextel.org

BUDDHIST MEDITATION & PHILOSOPHY

Mindfulness in Plain English (Bhante Henepola Gunaratana)
One of the most well-known and easy-to-read books on Mindfulness and Vipassana.

Wherever You Go There You Are: Mindfulness Meditation in Daily Life (John Kabat-Zinn)
A highly accessible book about Mindfulness Meditation in its secular form.

Turning the Mind into an Ally (Sakyong Mipham Rinpoche)
A great introduction to Buddhist meditation.

The Heart of the Buddha's Teaching: Transforming Suffering into Peace, Joy, and Liberation (Thich Nhat Hanh)
A modern overview of the teachings and practice of classical Buddhism.

Stages of Meditation (The Dalai Lama)
An overview of Buddhist meditation practices.

The Mind Illuminated (John Yates PhD)
A modern classic in the world of Buddhist meditation, emphasizing concentration practice.

Loving-Kindness: The Revolutionary Art of Happiness (Sharon Salzberg)
Focuses on Loving-Kindness Meditation and related practices.

Finding the Still Point: A Beginner's Guide to Zen Meditation (John Daido Loori)
A short introduction to Zazen.

Zen Mind, Beginners Mind: Informal Talks on Zen Meditation and Practice (Shunryu Suzuki)
An inspirational book on Zen practice and philosophy. Perhaps the most famous Zen book written in the last century.

The Compass of Zen (Seung Sahn)
A great overview of Zen.

Opening the Hand of Thought: Foundations of Zen Buddhist Practice (Kosho Uchiama Roshi)
This book gives you a real feel of the Zen practice of Just Sitting (*shikantaza*).

Dhamma.org
Vipassana meditation teachings by S.N. Goenka.
dhamma.org

Insight Meditation Society
Website of the Insight Meditation Society. Contemporary teachings and retreats on Vipassana, Mindfulness, and Loving-Kindness meditations. dharma.org

Access to Insight
An online library of traditional Buddhist texts and audios by teachers from the Thai forest tradition of Theravada Buddhism.
accesstoinsight.org

Tara Brach
Tara Brach's teachings blend Western psychology and Eastern spiritual practices. She is a well-known Buddhist teacher who also holds a PhD in Clinical Psychology.
tarabrach.com

Tricycle Magazine
The number one Buddhist magazine in the West.
tricycle.org

Zen Buddhism
One of the main websites on Zen Buddhism. Based on the Japanese Soto Zen tradition, this has a lot of resources for you to deepen your Zazen practice.
zen-buddhism.net

Audio Dharma
A library of free Buddhist teachings in audio format, by Insight Meditation Society teachers.
audiodharma.org

TAOIST MEDITATION & PHILOSOPHY

Tao: The Watercourse Way (Allan Watts)
A contemporary overview of the philosophy and practice of Taoism.

The Daodejing of Laozi (trans. Philip J. Ivanhoe)
The main text of Taoists, by the founder Laozi (Lao Tzu). Cryptic, deep, and poetic.

The Book of Chuang Tzu (trans. Martin Palmer)
A classic title presenting the teachings of Chuang Tzu, a main disciple of the founder of Taoism.

365 Tao: Daily Meditations (Deng Ming-Dao)
A more accessible book, with daily Taoist contemplations.

The Root of Chinese Qigong: Secrets of Health, Longevity, and Enlightenment (Dr. Yang, Jwing-Ming)
An in-depth overview of the history, theory, and practices of Qigong.

Inside Zhan Zhuang (Mark Cohen)
A book about the Tai Chi "Standing Like a Tree" meditation.

Taoistic
Your go-to source of online philosophical teachings on Taoism.
taoistic.com

SUFI MEDITATION & PHILOSOPHY

Sufism: The Transformation of the Heart (Llewellyn Vaughan-Lee PhD)
A great introduction to the philosophy and practice of Sufism.

Sufi Meditation and Contemplation (ed. Scott Kugle)
Contains a translation and commentary on three important Sufi texts, and is one of the most important books on the topic of Sufi meditation.

The Sufi Science of Self-Realization: A Guide to the Seventeen Ruinous Traits, the Steps to Discipleship, and the Six Realities of the Heart (Shaykh Muhammad Hisham Kabbani)
An important text outlining the Sufi path of spiritual purification and self-transformation.

The Healing Power of Sufi Meditation (Nurjan Mirahmadi as-Sayyid)
Although technical, it offers good and authentic information on Sufi methods.

The Essential Rumi (Jalal al-Din Rumi)
A collection of beautiful poems by the most famous Sufi of all times.

Living from the Heart (Puran Bair and Susanna Bair)
Describes a modern adaptation of Sufi Heartbeat Meditation, which focuses on syncing the breath with the heartbeat.

Sufi Saints & Sufism
In-depth exploration of the many spiritual practices of Sufism.
sufisaints.net

BIBLIOGRAPHY

While every effort has been made to ensure that the materials in this book are accurate, the publisher apologizes for any errors or omissions and would be grateful to be notified about any corrections. Sources are given in order of appearance across the spreads.

22–23 Sharpening your powers
F. Zeidan et al, "Mindfulness meditation improves cognition: Evidence of brief mental training", *Consciousness and Cognition* 19, no. 2 (2010), pp.597–605; L. S. Colzato et al, "Meditate to create: The impact of focused-attention and open-monitoring training on convergent and divergent thinking", *Frontiers in Psychology* 3, no. 116 (2012); B. K. Hölzel et al, "Mindfulness practice leads to increases in regional brain gray matter density", *Psychiatry Research: Neuroimaging* 191, no. 1 (2011), pp.36–43; P. Lush et al, "Metacognition of intentions in mindfulness and hypnosis", *Neuroscience of Consciousness* (2016), pp.1–10; P. Kaul, et al, "Meditation acutely improves psychomotor vigilance, and may decrease sleep need", *Behavioral and Brain Functions* 6, no. 47 (2010); E. Luders, et al, "The unique brain anatomy of meditation practitioners: Alterations in cortical gyrification", *Frontiers in Human Neuroscience* 6, no. 34 (2012).

24–25 The key to emotional wellbeing
F. Raes et al, "School-Based Prevention and Reduction of Depression in Adolescents: A Cluster-Randomized Controlled Trial of a Mindfulness Group Program", *Mindfulness* 5, no. 5 (2014), pp.477–486; A. J. Arias et al, "Systematic Review of the Efficacy of Meditation Techniques as Treatments for Medical Illness", *The Journal of Alternative and Complementary Medicine* 12, no. 8 (2006), pp.817–832; K. W. Chen, et al, "Meditative therapies for reducing anxiety: A systematic review and meta-analysis of randomized controlled trials", *Depression and Anxiety* 29, no. 7 (2012), pp.545–562; B. L. Fredrickson, et al, "Open Hearts Build Lives: Positive Emotions, Induced Through Loving-Kindness Meditation, Build Consequential Personal Resources", *Journal of Personality and Social Psychology* 95, no. 5 (2008), pp.1045–1062; J. S. Mascaro et al, "Compassion meditation enhances empathic accuracy and related neural activity", *Social Cognitive and Affective Neuroscience* 8, no. 1 (2013), pp.48–55; B. K. Hölzel et al, "Mindfulness practice leads to increases in regional brain gray matter density", *Psychiatry Research: Neuroimaging* 191, no. 1 (2011), pp.36–43; J. D. Creswell et al, "Mindfulness-Based Stress Reduction Training Reduces Loneliness and Pro-Inflammatory Gene Expression in Older Adults: A Small Randomized Controlled Trial", *Brain, Behavior, and Immunity* 26, no. 7 (2012) pp.1095–1101.

26–27 The Zen your body needs
J. Gu et al, "How do mindfulness-based therapy and mindfulness-based stress reduction improve mental health and wellbeing?", *Clinical Psychology Review* 37 (2015), pp.1–12; E. Epel et al, "Can meditation slow rate of cellular aging? Cognitive stress, mindfulness, and telomeres", *Longevity, Regeneration, and Optimal Health Integrating Eastern and Western Perspectives* (2009), pp.34–35; R. J. Davidson et al, "Alterations in brain and immune function produced by mindfulness meditation", *Psychosomatic Medicine* 65, no. 4 (2003), pp.564–570; M. Goyal et al, "Meditation Programs for Psychological Stress and Well-being: A Systematic Review and Meta-analysis", *JAMA Internal Medicine* 174, no. 3 (2014), pp.357–368; D. W. Orme-Johnson and V. A. Barnes, "Effects of the transcendental meditation technique on trait anxiety: A meta-analysis of randomized controlled trials", *The Journal of Alternative and Complementary Medicine* 20, no. 5 (2014), pp.330–341; R. H. Scheider et al, "Stress Reduction in the Secondary Prevention of Cardiovascular Disease", *Circulation: Cardiovascular Quality and Outcomes* 5, no. 6 (2012); M. Teut et al, "Effectiveness of a mindfulness-based walking programme in reducing symptoms of stress – a randomized controlled trial", *European Journal of Integrative Medicine* 4, no. 1 (2012), p.78.

INDEX

Page numbers in **bold** refer to main entries.

INDEX

INDEX

ACKNOWLEDGMENTS

ABOUT THE AUTHOR

Giovanni Dienstmann is not a guru nor a spiritual master, but a practitioner on the way, sharing the powerful tools, insights, and inspiration that have helped him in his own journey of personal growth and spiritual awakening.

Over two decades, Giovanni has tried more than 80 different meditation techniques, read over 200 books on the subject, and meditated for over 8,000 hours, and has spent time with Zen masters, monks, and Yogis from all over the world.

Now a meditation teacher, author, and coach, Giovanni seeks to translate and "update" the tools and teachings of worldwide wisdom traditions so they are easily digestible for the 21st-century person, with a systematic, non-sectarian, rational, and pragmatic approach. Giovanni shares his work on his website, LiveAndDare, which has been ranked in the top 5 meditation blogs in the world.

AUTHOR'S ACKNOWLEDGMENTS

I would like to make public my gratitude towards all the masters and teachers that have either directly taught me, or inspired me through their work.

Some names worth mentioning, among the ones I have personally met: Lakshmana Swami, Shivarudra Balayogi, Mooji, Joshin Sensei, Moriyama Roshi, Swami Muktibodhananda.

Some masters and figures that I haven't met, but who deeply influenced my development in the contemplative path, are: Ramana Maharshi, Shivabalayogi, Nisargadatta Maharaj, Papaji, Swami Satyananda, Swami Rama, Swami Vivekananda, Annamalai Swami, Sadhu Om, David Godman, David Frawley, Daniel de Ávila, Osho, Uchiyama Roshi, Adi Shankra, and the Buddha.

Last but not least, my expression of gratitude to Sepide Tajima, for all the caring support throughout my path of learning and teaching – including the patience with my obsessions, weird experiments, blindspots, and stubbornness.

PUBLISHER'S ACKNOWLEDGMENTS

The publisher would like to thank Keith Hagan for the jacket illustration, Louise Brigenshaw and Jade Wheaton for design assistance, Megan Lea, Rona Skene, and Alastair Laing for editorial assistance, Corinne Masciocchi for proofreading, Margaret McCormack for the index, Emily Reid from the Media Archive, Robert Dunn in Production, Lori Hand, and last but not least, US editor Kayla Dugger.